SOUL REALIZED
Unlocking the Sacred Keys to Becoming a Divine Human

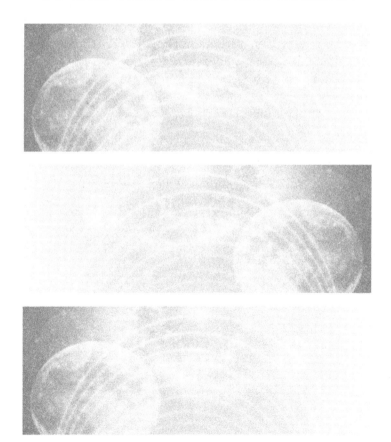

SOUL REALIZED
Unlocking the Sacred Keys to Becoming a Divine Human

by Meg Benedicte

Published by Quantum Healing Center, Inc.
1467 Siskiyou Blvd, #280
Ashland, OR 97520

Orders www.newearthcentral.com

All rights reserved. No part of this book may be reproduced or transmitted in any form or by any means, electronic or mechanical, including photocopying, recording or by any information storage and retrieval system, without written permission from the author, except for the inclusion of brief quotations in a review.

Copyright © 2010 by Meg Benedicte First Edition, January 2010
Second Edition, October 2016

Published in the United States

Edited by Robin Quinn, www.writingandediting.biz

Cover & Interior book design by James Arneson,
www.jaadbook design.com

SOUL REALIZED
Unlocking the Sacred Keys to Becoming a Divine Human

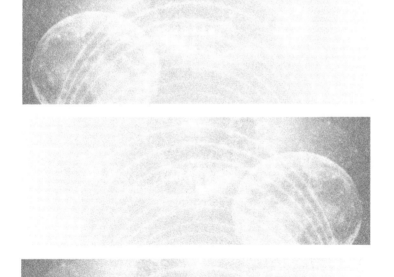

Meg Benedicte
Founder of Quantum Access™

I am eternally grateful to all my clients of the past two decades who have opened their hearts and shared their stories, for I would not be here without them.

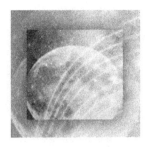

Table of Contents

Chapter One
AN AWAKENING • *1*

Chapter Two
WORLD OF DUALITY • *11*

Chapter Three
THE HUMAN ENERGY FIELD • *21*

Chapter Four
THE ORIGINAL DIVINE HUMAN • *29*

Chapter Five
THE HOLOGRAPHIC MIND • *37*

Chapter Six
THE SHADOW SELF • *45*

Chapter Seven
THE ENSLAVEMENT OF HUMANITY • *59*

Chapter Eight
VICTIM CONSCIOUSNESS • *67*

Chapter Nine
A CONTAINER OF LIGHT • *77*

Chapter Ten
SOUL RETRIEVAL • *89*

Chapter Eleven
A BRIDGE TO A NEW EARTH • *99*

SACRED SYMBOLS • *109*
SACRED GEOMETRY • *113*
GLOSSARY • *117*
REFERENCES • *121*
ABOUT THE AUTHOR • *123*

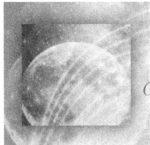

Chapter One

AN AWAKENING

MY STORY IS an unusual one, in that I am not able to relate to the life prior to my awakening. I do remember that it was a life filled with complexity, uncertainty and deep-seeded fear and sadness. The first year of life was in grave danger of being cut short as the physical body lay dying in a Los Angeles hospital due to complications from internal bleeding. Through remote viewing I see the hospital room and the faces of the adoptive parents peering through the oval window in the door.

The original incarnation was going to shift as my celestial Soul intercepted the fading body and claim the karmic life plan as my own. This was my Soul's new physical reality, my entry point into the earth plane and the first initiation of my life's mission.

I chose this particular incarnation for specific reasons. The first being the reptilian hybrid genetic codes inherited from the birth parents, and secondly, the ancestral lineage of my adoptive family's Ritual Abuse Program. Both of these elements provided access to dark, corrupted systems long held to oppress and control human consciousness. This particular human life plan was selected with care and precision so that I could pursue the primary purpose of my earthly visit – to intercept and dismantle the human prison of enslavement. I am here on a mission of intervention.

And so I have lived most of my life standing on the sidelines, observing human behavior and the established belief systems. I've always been conscious on some level that I didn't fit in, and I felt alone and abandoned here. It has taken half a century to acknowledge and accept that I am a visitor ... that I process information and respond differently than other beings. I recognize the value of all my observations and have been able to assemble and organize data in a comprehensive manner to be presented and shared for spiritual growth and evolution. As a celestial Time Jumper, I have less interference with the super-conscious mind and am able to pierce through the veils of illusion, and unconsciousness amnesia. This enables me to discern what exists in all dimensions of life. I have been straddling the world of material form and the unseen world of energy, drawing conclusions from all that I see, feel and hear in both worlds. This is not how human beings normally think, and it may surprise you to read what truly exists and is occurring in the planetary realm people live in. My focus and intention in sharing this information is to awaken and uplift all life on this planet into a world of Love, Union and Wholeness.

> "God can dream a bigger dream for you than you can dream for yourself, and your role on Earth is to attach yourself to that divine force and let yourself be released to it."
>
> • Oprah Winfrey

It has been a long journey getting here, but humanity has reached another turning point in history, a climactic time of karmic retribution, and we can influence the outcome. Can you sense it? Can you feel the shifts of consciousness happening, like shifting tides or the wind repositioning our future in a new direction? All of life is being affected by the quickening movement into a new reality, and we can flow with it or fight it. The choice is ours to make at this time.

Activating the Spiritual Energy

In a surprising turn of events, I experienced a powerful kundalini activation that culminated in a spiritual awakening of my Soul's lineage and purpose.

It was January 17, 1994 and the devastating Northridge Earthquake hit Los Angeles at 4:55 am ... I was jolted awake from a deep sleep by the massive earthquake, which sent ripples of lightening-strike energy down through my nervous system and into my cells. The catastrophic shock waves rippled through my body and unleashed a tidal wave of kundalini electrical force up my spine and into the hypothalamus in my brain. Not only did this awaken within me a higher awareness of human destiny, but it jolted an activation of new Soul energy to enter my physical body.

> "Soul appears when we make room for it."
> • Thomas Moore

I staggered out of bed and felt my way through the dark, going downstairs to the street, where I sat huddled in my robe on the curb in a transcendent daze. For several hours, my mind and body went through concentric shifts of consciousness, peeling away layers and layers of illusions of ego-identity and released blocked memory.

As my celestial Soul walked into the previous incarnation, awareness poured into my conscious mind and I never saw the world through the same eyes again! Out of the darkness, I began to "see" visions of the past, the present and the possible future. I recognized my Soul spark originated from Metatron's soul family, and my human reality was destined and purposeful. In the early hours of the earthquake's aftershocks, my whole bioenergetic system was pummeled with powerful kundalini activations ... shaking awake my understanding of the current human condition, the Matrix simulation and the ever-increasing transformation of human consciousness. In a true moment of clarity, I realized that the Age of Enlightenment was upon us!

My Initiation to the Quantum Vortex

In 1997, I experienced another initiation during a channeled reading with a gifted visionary. During trance states I saw my OverSoul as a celestial alchemist. Over the years, I began to communicate regularly with the Council of the 12 Tribes of the Great Central Sun and the elders of the Sirian High Council to gain better understanding of the current planetary Ascension Plan.

I was instructed to activate a spinning Vortex of Energy around my body, and to anchor it into my energetic field. They chuckled and suggested I bring a chair with me, for I would be working in this Vortex for a long time to come. Awkwardly, I proceeded to test the mechanics of living, breathing and manipulating energy while a funnel of light spun counter-clockwise around me. Many a morning, I would step out of bed and collapse in a heap, unable to stabilize the vertigo. But over time, as I practiced and tested the swirling movement, I began to recognize how *this amazing and powerful Quantum Vortex was the template of transformation in our Universe.*

Understanding the Science of Creation

Over the years, I began to gain a better understanding of the evolving science of creation being debated among physicists. According to quantum physicists, the Universe we live in resembles a sea of motion—a quantum field of vibrant activity. All matter in the Universe is interconnected by waves of energy that spread out through time and space, so that every part of the Universe is touching every other part instantaneously in a unified field of ether. These waves oscillate through space, like ripples on a pond, as carriers of information. It is the field we originate from, and the field to which we will ultimately return.

Astronomers have documented the natural movement of this Universal field as a spiraling whirlpool—visible in the swirling galaxies in space. Recent studies and in particular the Hubble cosmological data now show that the Milky Way Galactic Core is a massive black hole spinning at approximately the velocity of light. Mounting evidence supports the "black hole creation model"—demonstrating the Universal origin of galactic and stellar formation at the Galactic Center. NASA scientists have coined the phrase "co-evolution" to describe the phenomenon of combining sparks of crystalline light in spinning vortices (black holes) as Source Creation to birth new stars.

All of life in our dynamic Universe emerges from that single pulse of light, a multi-dimensional scalar standing wave pattern. Within the vacuum state of the Quantum Vortex beats the standing scalar wave of Singularity…the continual pulse of collapse and expansion of creation. It is the natural rhythm of life, like a cosmic heartbeat that fuels our Universe. There is growing astrophysical evidence that the vacuum structure found within galactic black holes also exists at the atomic scale level in our cells.

Faith is the strength by which a shattered world shall emerge into the light.

• Helen Keller

In May 2011 NASA headquarters announced the extraordinary results of their Gravity Probe-B mission…the data confirmed Einstein's predicted theory of relativity. They discovered a space-time Vortex spinning counter-clockwise around Earth! After a year of gathering data and 5 years of analysis, the NASA team was able to demonstrate that space and time are woven into a 4th dimensional fabric that curves clockwise around our planet, causing the "drag" of gravity.

Max Planck, a German physicist who is viewed as the Founding Father of Quantum Theory, discovered that subatomic particles never are at rest, but are reacting to the empty space around them. This creates a vibrant magnetic force at zero gravity that radiates energy. It has been calculated that the total energy of the Zero Point Field exceeds all energy in matter by a factor of 10^{40}.

In the fascinating book, *The Field: The Quest for the Secret Force of the Universe*, journalist Lynne McTaggart investigates this mysterious, inexhaustible energy source. "Attempts to extract energy from the Zero Point Field as an exotic means of aerospace travel, once the object of secret projects funded by modest seed money, have now been lavishly underwritten by corporate giants such as Lockheed Martin. The ultimate source of energy appears to be the zero-point radiation of the vacuum continuum."

In recent years, international laboratories have studied the vacuum effect of the Zero Point Field, or, for example, the stillness observed within spinning tornadoes. There is growing astrophysical evidence, substantiated by Swiss-born Nassim Haramein and his research team of physicists, electrical engineers, mathematicians and other scientists of the Resonance Project Foundation, in their published paper "Scale Unification: A Universal Scaling Law for Organized Matter."

Haramein's years of research uncovered evidence of the capacity of ancient civilizations' greater physics and mathematical understandings and engineering technology to control the gravitational fields required to build the pyramids in Egypt. "Technology that directly interacts with the vacuum," he claims, "directly interacts with the Source of Creation."

Buried deep within these ancient cultures are books of knowledge, sacred texts and practiced rituals that taught the chosen initiates mastery of advanced physics, utilizing the lost crystal-based technology once called the Arc of the Covenant. The students learned how to activate small-scale singularity, or mini-black hole power, to tap into the unlimited energy of the Quantum Vortex. In so doing, inspired by the secret wisdom of the Ancient Mystery Schools of Egypt, they dedicated their lives to attaining *Apotheosis*—the ultimate divine transformation of man into god! Originally from ancient Greek theology: *apo*—'to become', *theos*—'god'.

Learning the Ancient Sacred Wisdom

Following the same path that the ancient initiates discovered centuries ago, I began endless hours of experimentation. In the process, I learned that by applying Vortex energy to our human energy field, mimicking how the Universal ecosystem evolves, we can transform our own human existence. As our ancestors before us, we are discovering anew once-lost knowledge of the ancient mystery of Apotheosis in our quest to ascend into divinity. By tapping into the *phi* spin momentum of Black Hole dynamics in space, we are able to integrate Soul Energy inwards and release incongruent energy outwards. In the same manner, step by step, I began to transform my own human energetics and molecular structure. This extraordinary discovery was the inspiration for developing my proprietary healing process, Quantum Access™.

A little more background ... the Quantum Theory of Entanglement demonstrates that once subatomic particles are in contact, they influence each other in the same way no matter how far they are separated. This feature of "nonlocality" in quantum particles is seen in the case of identical twins who are separated at birth and yet still retain physical and behavioral similarities and telepathic connection. In this manner, we can see the human brain operates as a radio receiver and transmitter of quantum signals in a Unified Field of consciousness.

> Where love rules, there is no will to power and where power predominates, love is lacking. The one is the shadow of the other.
> ● Carl G. Jung

Over the following months and years, I trained my mind to access ancient knowldge, the stored cellular memory and akashic records on how to use the Quantum Vortex to heal myself. And so began several decades of spiritual pursuit, an ambitious race against time, to unlock my full potential while living in a dualistic world of separation. I had uncovered the untapped power for human transfiguration and unlocked the communication network to Universal intelligence. And so my personal evolution had begun! Step-by-step, I discovered how to maneuver and perform quantum transformation while spinning in the Vortex. Over the past decade, I had to continually stretch my human capacity to accelerate the expanding velocity and volume of a multi-dimensional spacetime continuum. I was compelled to run *phi* harmonic tones in my body to establish "order" in the subatomic particle field, so I could resonate like a tuning fork humming at the same frequency. I learned how to identify and invoke the harmonic frequency of *phi*, often called the Golden Ratio or Golden Proportion, as the means to balance and stabilize an error-free connection with the Zero Point Field.

The logarithmic spirals of the Quantum Vortex, as we see in the Whirlpool Galaxy, operate like fractals, whereby they are self-similar at all scales. Although the size of the spiral increases, the shape is unchanged with each successive swirl. Yet only those components at a particular resonance frequency in the fractal-like energy spectrum can manifest in the Quantum Vortex. By tuning in to the harmonic frequency of *phi* (Divine Proportion) within a logarithmic spiral, I was able to re-establish internal order, balance and stability—while metabolizing waves of photon light at the cellular level.

During my daily meditation practice in the Quantum Vortex, I disciplined my mental focus by staring at a candle flame, and eventually opened the inter-dimensional doorway of my mind. Lynne McTaggart's research reveals how our thoughts are focused ordered light acting like lasers—and "intentioned healing creates some of the most organized waves of light found in nature."

As I strengthened my mental muscle, I was able to remotely "tune in" and explore different places, people and events in a variety of locations in the past, present and future. This process, called Remote Viewing, is well documented in the book, *Cosmic Voyage*, as author Courtney Brown shares his personal experiences while participating in the U.S. government-funded psi (parapsychology) research sponsored by the Central Intelligence Agency (C.I.A.) and the Defense Intelligence Agency (D.I.A.).

My own research and discoveries laid the foundation for Remote Viewing and offering distance healing sessions to people all around the world. Not only could I interpret their energetic reality, but I also utilized the powerful Quantum Vortex to transform people's reality to match their destined Soul Purpose and Plan. Surrounded by the High Council and the clients' team of angels and guides, I began to uncover a shockingly hidden world of darkness, control and manipulation, and human genetic interference. Drawing from many years as an Energetic Surgeon and Seer, I was able to unlock the lost "holy grail" of creative manifestation and conscious transformation, piecing together the hidden truth of humanity's current condition. Over the past two decades, I have witnessed astonishing, mind-bending events with clients, as well as my own personal healing journey. I invite you to suspend all past preconceptions, as I uncover and share the mysteries of human history, the corrupted planetary hologram, and the coming Age of Enlightenment.

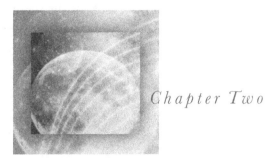

Chapter Two

WORLD OF DUALITY

WE ARE REACHING a time in human history when we are experiencing first-hand the effects of personal as well as collective karma. Meanwhile, our little planet exists within a spinning galaxy, surrounded by spacetime curvature providing continual feedback...even our DNA are spinning strands of genetic code! We are living in a bio-energetic organism designed to particulate matter according to the exchange of information streaming into the brain. And so all thoughts, emotions and actions that we experience are metabolized at certain frequencies into the brain and converted into our mind's perception of reality, just as our television set converts frequencies into a visual screen. Our brainwaves spin outward into the collective consciousness ... only to return and become our human reality.

We live in a 3rd-Dimensional World of Duality—a polarizing electro-magnetic force field of Light and Dark or positive/negative energy.

We are the living embodiment of Duality! For every positive action we take, there is an equal opposing force of negative reaction. This is the Principle of Duality – in an electromagnetic field opposite forces attract! The ever present balancing act of opposing, repelling forces of positive/negative magnetic states battle within our body, heart and mind. Physical matter is compressed between the gravitational forces of Polarization, or the orientation of wave oscillation pointing either positive or negative direction of the magnetic poles. Often misunderstood, the ever-present recurring resistance of negative or Dark forces is to be expected while living in the World of Duality. This is how our ecosystem retains balance and order within a polarized electro-magnetic field. It also explains why the Universal Law of Attraction is ineffective within a dualistic environment. Opposites attract within a polarized world!

> "How much longer will you go on letting your energy sleep? How much longer are you going to stay oblivious of the immensity of yourself?"
>
> • Bhagwan Shree Rajneesh

Not only did this become evident throughout my own life, but I continued to hear endless stories from my clients over the years of how counter-force was sabotaging all efforts to create, to manifest, and to evolve! A perfect example of this occurred in 2006, when received a series of visions and guidance from Spirit to collaborate and form a cooperative Healing Center in Los Angeles. My business partner found a beautiful site waiting for us next to a Yoga Center. We applied, were approved, and just needed to complete the final contract and move in. At the point of manifestation in the material world, the opposing force of Duality kicked in and sabotaged our Healing Center. The property owners gave empty promises, delayed the move-in date, and finally ignored our calls. The whole project "lost its legs" ... was no longer rooted in the material world. During this process, I could feel the incredible wave of counter-force pushing us backwards, opposing all forward movement to create something new. The field of Duality was sabotaging the Law of Attraction by opposing creative progress! According to the popular New Age film, *The Secret*, it is assumed that by utilizing the Law of Attraction we can proactively manifest the perfect identical match to our focused intention, visualization and energized feelings as electro-magnetic beings. Unfortunately, while living in a polarized environment, we only magnetize an opposing force that sabotages manifesting our dreams! It became apparent to me after years of countless efforts to manifest my Soul's purpose and destiny, that the only way to successfully manifest in the material world would require abandoning Duality and transition into living in the quantum field! I was determined to unlock the sacred key to enter a new world of Unity Consciousness and my transformational tool was the Quantum Vortex!

Overcoming Karma

The balancing system of a dualistic world is the Karmic Cycle, an eternal trap of polarized forces preventing human evolution. At the dawn of the 21st century, it is evident that we are currently in the grip of an extraordinary backlash of karmic energy! Not only is it extraordinary in its intensity, but it is deeply seeded within our planet's energetic body, erupting in natural disasters, wars, poverty, hunger and violence—affecting us all.

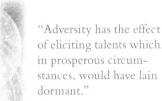

"Adversity has the effect of eliciting talents which, in prosperous circumstances, would have lain dormant."

• Horace

As long as we exist within an earth-bound human body, we will feel the ripples of karma continue to move through our psyche, our nervous system, and our biology. As the karmic wave builds in intensity, humanity is exhibiting more disease

> "A loving person lives in a loving world. A hostile person lives in a hostile world. Everyone you meet is your mirror."
> • Ken Keyes Jr.

in the physical, mental, emotional and spiritual realms.

How do we begin to heal the human karmic debt and reverse the damage to ourselves and to the planet? For we will never evolve until we can break free of this prison of polarized karma!

Our history as humans is also repeating itself! We sit and scratch our heads in perplexity and confusion, unable to digest the fact that we are on the brink of extinction once again. Everywhere we see signs of the wounded human psyche—fragmented minds brought on by the collapse of ancient mysticism, philosophy, science and human idealism, the onslaught of the Dark Ages and illiteracy and ignorance, and the increasing pressures of modern civilization. Will the global collective karma destroy another human civilization? What will it take for us to wake up and create a new earth?

The shift starts with each and every one of us owning our own personal karma and choosing to confront the depths of our personal Duality for healing. The capacity of the human ego's resistance to self-reflection, analysis and forgiveness is astonishing...but very real. We would rather distract ourselves with just about anything before we will confront our personal demons.

My Healing Journey

I came across this healing path as a direct response to my own debilitating patterns and wounded consciousness. At some point in my mid-thirties, I began to recognize that I had always attracted a certain type of man with similar behavior patterns as my adoptive father. On some conscious level, I felt like a human magnet for raging, cheating, abusive sexual addicts. My first course of treatment was traditional psychotherapy and Co-

Dependency Anonymous. But soon it became clear that I was dealing with a much deeper, darker, engrained force. I was caught in a swirl of karmic retribution and could not escape the hold it had on my life.

I've often heard, "Our deepest wounds lead us to our greatest gifts." By entering a heavily karmic incarnation, my Walk-In Soul was working through the previous owner's Soul Contracts, the entrapment of karma, and the suffering of human fragmentation. As a Soul Visitor, I had not built up karmic debt, and so this "life-swap" provided entry into the World of Duality and enabled me to viscerally learn about the current human condition.

"We must be willing to get rid of the life we've planned, so as to have the life that is waiting for us."

• Joseph Campbell

My life story propelled me into the awakening of Bio-Energetic Healing and the activation of the Quantum Vortex as my transformational tool. The pain, heartbreak and frustration fed my inner urgency to find a cure! Glimmers and glimpses of our beautiful human potential inspired me to break free of the prison holding me captive in my mind and body. I needed to resolve and eliminate the karmic debt and devote myself to the pursuit of self-realization.

Facing the Shadow Self

All of humankind is being offered the extraordinary opportunity to travel the path towards becoming a Divine Human, the physical embodiment of the Soul. That journey entails the gradual healing, clearing and releasing of all polarized negativity from our bodies, our auric fields, and our subconscious mind.

We must begin to observe and recognize our life lessons, as we reflect and analyze our personal patterns and behaviors. The key to unlocking karma is the wisdom it imparts as we allow ourselves to receive the soothing balm of forgiveness

> "Responsibility is not inherited, it is a choice that everyone needs to make at some point in their life."
>
> • Byron Pulsifer

and compassion. Wisdom erases all karma! Every aspect of human life has meaning and purpose ... we need to awaken out of our fragmented mental distractions, open our eyes to truth and become "The Observer".

As we delve deeper into our shadow self, we uncover the negatively charged areas ready for healing and forgiveness! Every layer of shadow that we probe, uncover, heal and integrate will contribute to the increased raising of our energetic vibration. As we let go of more and more heavy, dense, stuck energy, we begin to accelerate our energyfrequency and feel lighter and lighter. We experience lighter thoughts, lighter emotions, and also lighter bodies! By converting the dense, lower vibrational shadow consciousness of Duality into higher consciousness, we enhance our physical health and well-being. We begin to feel less disconnected and empty inside and more Soul presence and joy in our daily lives.

From Ego-Centered to Soul Consciousness

It's important to understand that we are not our minds. The lower egoic mind controls our human self and exists in Duality and 3D Time. Our lower mind is the less developed, almost child-like aspect of our personality. It only believes in what it can see, hear and touch in the physical world. The only way to break free of the limitations of the material plane is to step out of the ego mind's reality and begin to observe and address life from the higher perspective of the Soul. In his book *The Four Insights,* leading psychologist and medical anthropologist Alberto Villoldo, Ph.D. describes the nebulous concept of the Soul as "the best word we have for that essential part of ourselves that seems to have preceded our entry into this world, yet also endures after our lifetime."

There needs to be a shift in power, like the passing of a baton, from the controlling human ego to the wisdom of the timeless Soul in order to break free of Duality and evolve into becoming a Divine Human. This can be one of the most harrowing of experiences, often called the "dark night of the soul," when the ego resists change and battles to maintain control of the lower will and the earthly life. Unfortunately, the ego mind doesn't understand that it only exists in the physical plane and thus its decisions are limited and based only on what it can see, hear or touch. This is not a part of our personality that should be wielding power and influence in our lives!

We tend to blame outside forces when we don't get what we want, not realizing that everything is flowing into our lives as a result of our past actions. When we can move into following the wisdom of the Soul and feel the presence of our personal power and true essence, then we are able to take full responsibility for what we create in life. It is only when we shift our awareness and see through the "eyes of the Soul" that we can see the consequences of our past egoic decisions, actions and words. We are then able to own and accept the legacy of the less-developed self and begin the process of clearing the negative energy from the past, so that we can move into the purity of the future.

It is this process of "internal house-cleaning" that frees us from the shackles of the past, the locks and chains holding us frozen in the limitations of time. By cleaning out all shadow consciousness of the egoic self, we can break free of the limiting beliefs, patterns and programs that have kept us prisoners in Duality and move into the multi-dimensional pulse and stillness of Singularity. It opens the heart to feel the natural flow of abundance and the exquisite joy present in the quiet moments in life. As we disentangle from the dark web of Duality and break free of the Karmic Cycle, we can soar to the heights of our visions and feel the bliss of freedom.

*I*n summary, humanity exists in a devolving world of karmic debt and the ever-battling forces of Light and Dark. All efforts to manifest as creative beings (through the Law of Attraction) are sabotaged by the polarizing counter-force of Duality. The path to enlightenment requires the dismantling of Duality and ego-control so that we can dedicate our lives to the wisdom and purpose of the Soul.

Healing Exercises

Observations: Armed with the knowledge and awareness of Duality, we can begin to observe and witness the flow of opposing forces in our lives. By checking inside to how our energy feels, we can start to identify what energy feels positive in our lives and what energy is opposing the natural flow of life force. Opposition feels constricting, limiting and blocked. It can manifest in a variety of ways, the main objective being counter-force to block and stop positive growth and expansion. We see it as some kind of repeated sabotage pattern that limits and derails our positive intentions.

The path to freedom is realizing where Duality exists in our daily lives and removing it. We must first identify all patterns of thinking, emoting and behaving that are sabotaging our efforts to manifest our fullest potential. These can surface as feelings of insecurity, lack of confidence, low self-worth…or beliefs that prohibit our expansion. Some common polarizing belief systems are "I'm not good enough", "I don't have permission", "I'm on the outside" or "It will never work".

And then there is the opposing push-back we experience whenever we do press forward to create something new. We live in a geomagnetic field driven by north and south poles compressing everything with gravity. The balance point is always adjusting between the positive and negative energies. All positive action forward meets an equal negative reaction backwards. Take some time to watch, observe and analyze this continual polarized push-pull occurring in your daily life. This will illuminate where Duality is present and operating in your mind/body matrix.

1. Use the Quantum Vortex to collapse and clear all discordant thoughts, emotions, and patterns of dis-ease—and pulse alive your new healthy body, clear mind, joyful heart and calm Center.

2. Spinning in the Quantum Vortex accelerates the oscillation of our sub-atomic particles to **UNLOCK** and break free from the dense, polarized magnetic field that is keeping us stuck, unable to improve our life situation.

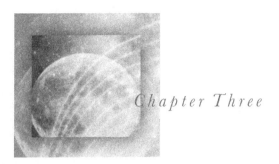

Chapter Three

THE HUMAN ENERGY FIELD

DURING THE EARLY years of working in the Quantum Vortex, I began to gain a clear understanding of how energy moves, undulates and influences the material world of form. I watched, observed and intuited the ebb and flow of energy between human beings, between humans and nature, and between the planets in our solar system. The very nature of our Universe is holistic, in that it is interrelated within a Grand Field of interlocking waves and particles of light, forming the ether lattice of collective consciousness. Even the Milky Way Galaxy resides within the macrocosm of this Unified Field, existing within a powerful field of potent creation.

In every particle of our being, we are connected to the infinite intelligence of the quantum field, or godhead. The very nature of our humanness allows access into the field of all possibilities. We must see ourselves as co-creators of our human existence, as our minds and bodies interact within the flowing abundance of Universal energy.

We are not separate "islands" existing in time, as our ego mind suggests, but human energy fields responding and transmitting consciousness all around us. According to Quantum Physics, the very act of observing and reacting to our environment penetrates the quantum field, and sets into motion an energetic exchange that influences the potential outcome.

Not only do humans exist within a powerful Universal Field of Energy, but our planet sustains a polarized field of opposing forces. As discussed in the last chapter, the existence of Duality, or field of polarized energy, affects the rhythm of forces within our own human reality. As holistic beings, we absorb the properties of the planetary electro-magnetic field as our operating system.

> "I am enough of an artist to draw freely upon my imagination. Imagination is more important than knowledge. Knowledge is limited. Imagination encircles the world."
>
> • Albert Einstein

Teetering in the balance point between positive and negative forces (Light and Dark), our human reality is a mirror reflection of our internal condition. We literally operate as a magnet, humming in a certain range of positive/negative frequencies. Once we realize that we are morphing and expanding in relation to the surrounding energy, we begin to recognize the impact of our thoughts, intentions and emotions as they flow into the mix. If all humans are energetic fields vibrating to a certain frequency of output, our mental and emotional state is directly affecting the condition of our environment. And vice versa!

After years of spinning my personal human energy field in the Quantum Vortex, I found that I could no longer ignore or give free reign to my subconscious thoughts or feelings, for they were directly affecting my human reality. If I was feeling insecure or judgmental, my interactions with others would become more difficult. If I was exhausted or not feeling nurtured, my business would slow down. If I was distracted or overwhelmed, I had accidents, dropped items, broke things.

If I became fearful or anxious, my heart would constrict and mymoney would disappear!

And so I had to learn to stay focused in the present moment, to act with loving care, and only give my attention and energy to what I valued. I had gradually become an integrated holistic being, and people, places and events were continually responding to my energetic output. I needed to start living as a Conscious Being!

Living in the Flow, or Not

As our energy field flows and responds to the surrounding planetary field, we can sense whether it has a positive or negative resonance frequency to our personal Soul energy signature. We are capable of perceiving the harmonic range or bandwidth with our internal sensory system, just like antennas picking up incoming radio frequency.

"I was there in the beginning and I was the spirit of love."
• Rumi

The foundation of the human energy body is composed of tiny wheels of light, or Chakra energy centers that provide access for incoming and outgoing "chi" or life force. Running through the center of our internal core is a vertical pillar anchoring the energetic vortices (chakras) that metabolize life force energy into our biology. Through the power of the breath, we direct energy to flow vertically up and down the pillar of chakras to replenish life force in our physical body. Our human energy field is designed like a tower of antennas positioned and pointed into the multiple levels or dimensions of our Universe.

When we are strongly rooted into our bodies, we have access to this amazing bio-circuitry and sensory system (chakra antenna tower) that can discern and distinguish the very nature of incoming energy. When our antenna receptors are disconnected from our bodies, we are deprived of a very sophisticated system of discernment, and we start to rely more heavily on the lower ego mind to make decisions and determine the direction of our lives.

Without the constant feedback from our Chakra sensory system, we are unable to navigate the unseen world of energy in daily decisions. Our thoughts and emotions cloud our clarity and the stresses of the day infringe on our natural ability to sense and intuit what is aligned with inner truth. Our ego mind continues to deconstruct the stream of incoming data from a handicapped position, blind to the powerful influence of Universal intelligence.

In this state, our decision-making process becomes dominated by the ego mind, which distrusts and rejects anything it cannot verify with the five physical senses. All incoming consciousness traveling in photon light from the quantum field is discarded as suspect and eventually shut off completely. By our very own minds, we are disconnected and separated from the powerful sensory system inherent to all of humanity.

Body/Mind/Spirit

Bio-Energetics is the study of the production of energy through respiration and metabolism, as well as determining where the flow of energy "chi" may be blocked, stagnant or contracted. Bio-Energetic Healing addresses the mind/body interaction and the subsequent healing therapy applied to repair, mend and reintegrate the powerful mind/body/spirit connection.

Based on Quantum Mechanics and Einstein's Unified Field Theory, throughout time, every thought, emotion, fear and belief is stored in our cellular structure. This eventually evolves into the blueprint that produces our 3rd-dimensional image in matter. The swirling strands of DNA code are the conveyors of genetic information that determine our entire physical existence; and this can be changed! By correcting the focused intention of our thoughts, like switching the channels on the television, we can transform the molecular patterning that creates our human experience.

The Flexibility of Time

Theoretical physicist Fred Alan Wolf, PhD, notes that "Buddha said he could move backward through time. Time travel is not just science fiction; it may actually be possible." In his book, *The Yoga of Time Travel,* Wolf interweaves the principles of yoga and Quantum Physics to show that time is a flexible projection of the mind. He explains how time and thought are bound together and why a change in ego structure could allow freedom from time's limitations. Wolf believes that "under certain circumstances, we might not only visit but even *alter* the past, with a ripple effect on the present."

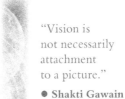

"Vision is not necessarily attachment to a picture."

● Shakti Gawain

The timeless Soul, our original Spark of Creation, experiences the entire spectrum of the human condition as multiple soul aspects existing simultaneously in different timelines. If there were ever any doubt in my mind about reincarnation, my healing practice working in the Quantum Vortex dispelled any question about death and rebirth.

The groundbreaking work by Brian L. Weiss, M.D., in *Many Lives, Many Masters,* introduced reincarnation and past-life regression to the mainstream. Dr. Weiss, a psychiatrist and Yale Medical School graduate, was surprised and compelled to learn more about reincarnation when his patients were able to describe detailed, verifiable memories of past-life experiences during hypnosis.

Deepak Chopra, author of *Ageless Body, Timeless Mind,* claims "it is our ability to break the illusion of linear time and experience a domain that is eternal, timeless, and acausal ... that helps conquer all fear including the fear of death and gives us a glimpse into the immortal nature of our soul." By spinning in the timeless, multi-dimensional Quantum Vortex, I was able to connect to my Soul's entire Field of Consciousness. At a glimpse, it appeared in the image of a wheel, the hub being the timeless Soul presence, and the spokes of the wheel being all the different timelines (incarnations) of reality. This reflects the concept that all the Soul's timelines exist simultaneously, but each timeline is being experienced as an individual soul "aspect" in a particular time and space continuum.

For example, my soul "aspect" that embodies Meg is living in the time and space coordinates of 1959 to now, in Los Angeles, California. But my Soul hub is feeding into every timeline (the wheel analogy) simultaneously. This is extraordinary for it enables us to connect to parallel timelines and adjust, heal or clear discordant energy and update the entire system (energy wheel) to the upgrade. Not only does this allow humanity to resolve and close out past-life karma, soul contracts, vows and trauma, but we can now heal and upgrade all of the soul timelines at once.

In summary, as holistic beings, our human energy field (mind/body/spirit) is constantly interacting with the Universal Field—a vibrant, responsive network of consciousness that mirrors our internal condition. Outside of the limitation of time, we can access past-lives to heal and transform our current life's direction and evolution.

Healing Exercise

Observations: In order to access the magnificent bounty of our spiritual essence, we must move beyond the limiting world view of self-absorption and into becoming the Witness of our daily lives. This requires learning how to step outside of being controlled by our mind and into living in Observer Consciousness.

We can develop this additional dimension of Self-Observation by quieting the mind in meditation, raising the frequency of brainwave activity, and documenting our random negative thoughts and feelings, dramatic battles and struggles, deep inner wounding, charged emotional reactions, and any roadblocks to manifesting our full potential in life!

1. Start a Journal and begin to jot down a running list of all examples that you observe are running through your mind or feeling in your body that prevent you from experiencing vibrant, joyful, empowering wholeness!

    a. Examples of Negative Thoughts; "I'm not good enough", "I'm not lovable", "I can't cope with this", "I can't make any money", "They are rejecting me", "They won't let me succeed"

    b. Examples of Negative Feelings; fear, anxiety, insecurity, low self-worth, feeling unattractive, feeling rejected, feeling victimized

2. Make a 'mental note' of all debilitating patterns, beliefs and emotional reactions that do not reflect your true essence. Awareness of our limitations is the first step in breaking free!

    a. Make a List of all observable patterns operating in your daily life that seem to be repeating over and over again.

    b. Examples of Sabotaging Patterns: attracting abusive friends and lovers, gossiping, excessive addictive behavior, emotionally withdraw in intimacy, cannot complete any project, promiscuity, grandiosity.

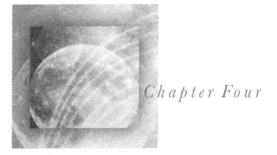

Chapter Four

THE ORIGINAL DIVINE HUMAN

IT'S BEEN SAID THAT human beings were created in the likeness of God/Goddess! This implies that our human genetic blueprint was designed as a holographic replica of Divine Creator. Well, I don't know about you, but humanity overall doesn't appear to be exhibiting many "God-like" qualities these days. If humans were originally created in the image of God/Goddess, what happened to degenerate the Divinity of humankind and how can we find our way back? How can we fulfill our destiny as Divine Humans?

These questions compelled my investigation into the root cause of our current human condition, as I demanded to be shown why we are in such poor shape and how can we realize our full potential again. I spent many hours time-traveling in the Quantum Vortex to remote view the history and orign of the human race. This provided a context for the true nature of the Original Human Prototype that was seeded by the 12 Tribes of the Great Central Sun

The Magnificence of the Divine Human

The qualities of the original 12th-dimensional human prototype were coded into packets of genetic material that responded to and were formed in union with focused intelligence. In a sense, human beings were designed to co-create their own physical manifestation in every moment. They were the perfect embodiment of Creation in every evolving reflection of conscious awareness and inspiration. They looked like a continually morphing life form in constant creative motion.

The human life form took on qualities of the Universal circuitry of energetic power—a pulsing, thriving extension of the rhythm of nature. As our physical bodies particulated into matter, they were encoded with a genetic framework for an artery network consisting of "ley lines" or pathways for Universal energy to flow through. The Human Energy Field was patterned on the Universal model of interlocking pathways as conduits of consciousness to travel between dimensional planes. Drawing from Gregg Braden's research on past mysticism and modern science in his book, *The Divine Matrix*, he has stated that "in 1944, Max Planck, the Father of Quantum Theory, shocked the world by saying that this 'matrix' is where the birth of stars, the DNA of life, and everything between originates...It is the missing link in our understanding that provides the container for the Universe, the bridge between our imagination and our reality, and the mirror in our world for what we create in our beliefs."

The orignal human race was designed as multi-dimensional life forms—open and receptive to Universal Intelligence. These 12th dimensional humans were able to transfer consciousness along the multi-dimensional bi-circuitry network as telepathic beings. Not only were they able to communicate amongst

> "Anything you do has a still point. When you are in that still point, you can perform maximally."
>
> • Joseph Campbell

The Original Divine Human

themselves, but their awareness was receptive to other life forms in the Universe. They were created in love, and were fueled by love. It was the very life force that sustained their human life forms. And so, the original human prototype was designed to exist and thrive on the energy of love. The packets of human genetic coding were engineered to metabolize the Universal energy of love as their food source.

The genetic blueprint for human life was designed to function as alchemical beings—a constantly responsive holographic imagery of light consciousness. And so, man/woman were not only coded to be able to survive on the energy of Creation, which is love, but also to be able to morph and manifest shape and form in a constant state of motion. We were not intended to be static beings of density.

> "This is the nature of genius, to be able to grasp the knowable even when no one else recognizes that it is present."
>
> • Deepak Chopra

Originally, human beings were designed to metabolize Light as a food source for growth and propagation. There was an endless stream of light energy pulsing in the quantum field that enabled the original humans to live on breath. It operated in similar fashion to photosynthesis in plant life. Our human genetic coding was designed to metabolize life force into the physical form from photon light particles. We were able to convert the energy of love in the light particles into fuel in the sub-atomic particles of the nucleus, and to maintain a constant in-flow of source energy from the interconnecting light network of the Unified Field. All of our needs were met by the quantum field around us!

In keeping with the totality of Creator Source, our human ancestors were complete, whole, the perfect embodiment of yin/yang union. The male/female connection provided the conduit for Light to travel through the bio-circuitry. As the original spark of creation from Creator Source, human ancestors were birthed as twin flame love in its totality. It was their natural state of being! They were designed as the perfect holographic reflection of the Godhead. The abundant Universe was their home, and they experienced the totality of all existence as their natural environment.

> "Intuition is the discriminative faculty that enables you to decide which of two lines of reasoning is right. Perfect intuition makes you a master of all."
>
> • Paramahansa Yogananda

The driving force of human genetic conception by the 12 Tribes, was the influx of Divine in telligence mapping through the timeless mind and conveyed as command code sequences into the physical receptor cells. There was an interlocking network of conscious direction from the mind to the human form, thus the introduction of "mind over matter." Very similar to how life is created in our Universe—consciousness could be made manifest! Humans were designed to operate as the Creator Source, by witnessing the holographic reflection materialize from their conscious inspiration.

And so, this begs the question—what happened? Why can't humans live like this anymore? And how do we return to our original Divine heritage again in the future?

Corrupted Beings

If we look at the current human condition now, we see a very different story. Our minds are dominated by the left brain, with limited access to the three dimensions of the material world, only trusting the five senses of physical reality. Our bodies are dense, solid matter, not alive with light particles. Our genetic coding has been manipulated to devolve and decay in the Time Matrix into eventual death. Human health is compromised by environmental bacterial and viral infectious disease, genetic mutation and diminished life force. We no longer reflect the holographic image of God/ Goddess!

In our current state, we use chemical pharmaceuticals to fight chronic conditions and surgery to cut out diseased human tissue. The modern medical experts view our human bodies as mechanical instruments that operate independently from our minds. The notion of a human Soul is scoffed at by our society at large, instead preaching a passive, victimized position of helplessness to a chaotic universe. Cultural religions encourage placing personal power in the hands of false gods, gurus or prophets. We were designed to be creator-gods ourselves! When did we switch to worshiping a power outside ourselves? How did we become so disempowered as humans?

"What is genius but the power of expressing a new individuality?"

• Elizabeth Barrett Browning

As I searched for clues while spinning in the timeless Quantum Vortex, I was able to trace the current human condition to the introduction of genetic manipulation and the subsequent reengineering of a hybridized human race.

As I "peered" into the conception of the holographic reality of the dual opposing spin of Duality centuries ago, it can be traced to the limiting double helix DNA of today. Clearly the original human race had somehow become tragically reduced in power, capacity, magnitude and position in the Universe. The human holographic imprint as the embodiment of Creator Source had been replaced with a shell of its original potential. The human mind had been intercepted and entrapped by a dark force.

Trapped in the Life/Death Cycle

There is much evidence of significant degradation of the genetic blueprint and the diminished capacity of the human race. In recent studies, theoretical physicists have developed the superstring theory which identifies zero-dimensional filaments of light, strings or membranes as the basic fundamental element of 11 dimensions in our Universe. The 12th dimension of divine connection was humanity's access (portal) to 'heaven on earth'. All that remains of the original 12-strand DNA is the double helix of duality, severely limiting humanity's ability to access and operate in all 12 dimensions of the Universe. The cellular corruption prevented access to the God Seed Code, now replaced with the mutated death code. Instead of living in perpetual creative motion, humans became trapped in a continual life/death karmic cycle of reincarnation.

Described in the Book of Genesis, the creation story of the Garden of Eden and the subsequent "Fall of Man" was humanity's first introduction to Duality. The Serpent, the reptilian symbol representing the seduction of evil, persuades Eve to taste of the Tree of Knowledge, saying that by doing so she and her mate could "be as gods, knowing good and evil." Adam, seeking external power and dominion, eats the fruit too. This is the first time we see humans reaching outside themselves to consume external energy (the apple).

The Creation story symbolizes the formation of the separate ego-identity now banished to a world polarized by the opposing existence of good and evil. Humanity has been caught in the downward spiral of human devolution into a constant state of ego-separation—keeping humankind in bondage and trapped in exile. The Original trauma of separation (Original Sin) remains deeply wounded in the human energy field, and perpetuates endless grief, sadness and despair in the inner spirit. If not resolved and healed, humanity cannot rise up out of the holographic prison of planetary enslavement. We will remain trapped in the life/death cycle of polarity, never free to ascend into our human lineage as multi-dimensional Divine beings.

In summary, the original human prototype was designed by the 12 Tribes of the Great Central Sun in the image of God/Goddess, the perfect embodiment of wholeness (yin/ yang) as a morphing, self-sustaining creative being. Since the "Fall of Man" and the insertion of Darkness, humankind has devolved into a polarized shell of lost potential, evident in the remaining corrupted (double helix) DNA and exile of ego-separation.

Healing Exercise

Intuition: Two of the most effective tools for opening your connection to psychic intuition is meditation and automatic writing. When you calm the incessant chatter in the mind and move into quiet, internal stillness, you can finally hear the soft, subtle guidance from your Higher Self. Humanity cannot ascend without daily meditation.

The Quantum Access™ technique will enhance your ability to create deeper connection in all four levels of your being – the physical, mental, emotional and spiritual. By working with sacred geometry, the templates of creation, you are opening the portal to higher dimensional consciousness and understanding. When combining the Quantum Access™ Activations with free-flowing channeled writing you are able to reconnect to the inner voice of Spirit.

1. Set time aside early in the morning or before bed to create a sacred space for meditation and unrestrained writing – this will open up the connection between the higher mind of Spirit and the lower mind of your human self.

2. Try not to audit the words written – just record all thoughts as they flow through your mind. Not only will you gain a better understanding of the repetitive negative thought forms of the less developed Ego, but you start to open to higher consciousness as well. Tune inside and become an open channel to Spirit!

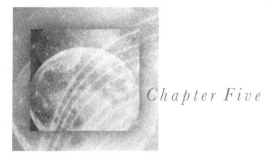

Chapter Five

THE HOLOGRAPHIC MIND

SOME YEARS AGO, while working in the Quantum Vortex, I was guided by the High Council to upgrade how I ground my human energy field onto Earth. I was instructed to unlock my field from the polarized 3D Earth grid, or meridian lines running in the planet, for they had become corrupted. As you can imagine, I became alarmed, and so began my investigation into the current condition of our planet's dualistic nature.

Step-by-step I was guided to anchor my feet and root my energy field onto the bottom platform of my aura, secured onto the 5th dimensional crystalline global grid. In a very real sense, I was about to move "off the grid." I pulled out, adjusted the chakra magnets on my feet, and began a gradual process of securing a contained human energy field into a higher frequency 5D field.

An Amazing Capability Lost

There has been much scientific research on how our minds are able to influence our external world reality. The human mind operates like a movie projector and the inner eye streams images outward as though through the lens of a camera (our 3rd Eye Chakra). This continual stream of consciousness creates an array of ideas, visions, beliefs and judgments that propel forth like laser light into the quantum field and forms our holographic reality.

> "True silence is the rest of the mind; it is to the spirit what sleep is to the body, nourishment and refreshment."
> • William Penn

As described in *The Hidden Messages in Water,* Dr. Masaru Emoto discovered that different conditions and different thoughts directed at frozen water influenced the crystals within it. Water from pristine springs or water exposed to "loving words" revealed snowflake patterns that were "brilliant, complex, and colorful." On the other hand, water that was polluted, or exposed to "negative" thoughts formed "incomplete, asymmetrical patterns with dull colors." Emoto reports that the molecules of water are impacted by "our thoughts, words and feelings."

If the human mind determines how our reality materializes, then it becomes essential that human beings learn how to master their own flow of consciousness. Without discernment, the human mind's creative powers could be misused. This begs the question, what if an outside presence could program human minds to create a world reality of limited consciousness and robotic-like behavior? What if humanity actually existed in an artificial holographic model of illusion that was dominated and manipulated by an external controlling force? What if our mind was being programmed by an artificial computer simulation that blocks our inherent intelligence and personal power?

Manipulation & Mind Control

Through a series of visions and remote viewing, I discovered just how distorted and debilitated the earthly reality had become over the past centuries since the "Fall of Man."

I began to uncover a surprising holographic insertion of manipulation and mind-control that humanity has been entrapped in. It appears that the earth plane has been invaded and controlled by a ruling ET race who owns the majority of wealth, land and political power.

It led me on a journey back in time to the initial conception of a mastermind plan of mind control and genetic re-engineering that would shift the positions of power. By inserting a holographic Time Matrix into the collective, all human evolution would cease and become stuck in the polarized fluctuations of positive/negative reactions.

"Life reflects your own thoughts back to you."

● Napoleon Hill

As the airways flooded the human brain/mental body with debilitating belief systems and separation consciousness, a perceptible decline in cognitive awareness and spiritual connection occurred. Increasingly we were operating in the downward spiral of human disease, decay and eventually death ... drained of our very life force and inner Spirit.

An Artificial Mind Matrix

During Quantum Access™ sessions with clients, I investigated this inserted human Mind Matrix. It appears like a series of frequency fences or interlocking walls of a complex maze, blocking full cognition in the mind. It is a closed system that locked human souls in the astral plane. The portal for Soul entry into earthly incarnations had been commandeered and human souls were being redirected into this illusory holographic system and unable to transition back to Source Creator.

As human souls incarnated, their re-engineered genetics entrapped them in a controlled earth plane while the reptilian brain stem was manipulated with mind-control programming.

Eventually human minds and bodies experienced psychic attack, separation consciousness, and depletion of Spiritual life force.

Upon the collapse of the Atlantian civilization, the gatekeepers of this bio-energetic technology spread to outlying territories, including ancient Egypt and pagan Britain. We see the declineof both cultures, as well as a slow erosion of the ancient teachings of the Egyptian Mystery Schools and the mysticism of the Goddess in Avalon. History paints a picture of the rising power of the dominant patriarchal hierarchy of Vatican Rome, and the gradual demise of the "Fall of Man" into the Dark Ages.

> "In this holographic world, everyone is you and you are always talking to yourself."
> • Debbie Ford

Immediately from birth, human souls would connect and interact with the Time Matrix simulation: their subconscious mind being fed an endless stream of divisive and destructive consciousness that separated them from their Divine lineage and divine Soul presence.

The artificial Mind Matrix streams debiliating programming into the family of origin, religions, cultural and societal dictates and mores, as well as the media—polluting the airwaves and controlling the subconscious mind. The simulation software develops a shadow Ego-identity that controls our lives, and asserts its will in opposition to Spiritual growth and change. This Ego implant is the source of resistance that we experience when we try to surrender to the wisdom of the Soul.

The Ego mind is a false identity deeply engrained and controlled by the polarizing "victim-persecutor" program, which is divisive in nature. It is the very opposite of what we need to evolve and ascend into Divine Humans.

The Addiction Cycle

Another major challenge facing humanity is the addiction program. It invades our being in myriad ways. Basically it is programming us to crave energy outside our selves, becoming obsessed parasitic consumers. It's extremely effective in separating us from our internal source of life force and Divinity. We are programmed to feed on other people's energy in relationships—a condition called "co-dependency." We are escaping and numbing ourselves with addictions to substances that heighten endorphins—such as drugs, alcohol, sugar, coffee, spending money, sex, adrenaline, etc.

Addictive patterns develop in early childhood as a coping mechanism to the ever-present darkness of Duality and the absence of unconditional love. The Ego mind separates us into isolation, emptiness, loneliness, a "me against the world" consciousness, and then we use addictions to fill the empty hole inside. What a vicious cycle to become entrapped in! It is truly an ingenious way to keep humanity disempowered and easily manipulated.

"If you admire greatness in another human being, it is your own greatness you are seeing."

• Debbie Ford

Why is this so effective? Observe how you feel when you experience being attacked. First you feel hurt, deeply wounded, in pain, betrayed and rejected. You feel victimized by the attacker, which then eventually leads to the feelings of anger, rage and revenge building up inside. At this point, the Matrix has entrapped us. We are now swinging back and forth between feeling the pain of victimization or avenging rage (becoming persecutors ourselves).

This destructive cycle pulls humanity down into deeper and darker emotions, building into a powerful quagmire of negatively charged toxic emotional energy! The cycle becomes stuck looping in the mind and pulsing in the emotional body. We become fragmented, split out of union, and go out of balance and into separation. As we continually swing between the victim-persecutor identities, we witness the gradual destruction of our human energy field and human spirit.

As our self-esteem is crushed and our confidence erodes, the persecutor identity develops into the Ego personality. The polarity of "greater than/lesser than" takes hold within the human psyche—the broken spirit feels "less than" and the grandiose Ego believes it is "greater than" everything. The Ego becomes hyper-critical, judgmental, rejecting, attacking and obsessed with "a service to self" lifestyle. The Ego has embodied the shadow presence of the persecutor polarity.

At this point, the holographic mind has become enslaved within the 3D Time Matrix and continues to aggressively assert dominance over human life. As the persecutor program takes hold, the human mind projects and asserts its self-indulgent will and agenda for control, consumption and pleasure. We have become slaves to our shadow side, and separated from our Divine Essence.

---

*I*n summary, the human mind projects a continual stream of consciousness that creates an array of ideas, visions, beliefs and judgments that propel forth like laser light into the quantum field and forms our holographic reality. Self-mastery involves observing, evaluating and reprogramming the nature of our holographic projections to better reflect our true Soul essence.

Healing Exercise

Vision Board: One of the most elusive aspects of human evolution and self-actualization is deciphering your soul purpose in life. How can you begin to know your Soul truth if you cannot even maintain Soul Presence in your body/heart/mind? True knowledge comes from personal experience! By using Quantum Access™ regularly you can eliminate polarity in your Human Energy Field and pull more and more Soul energy into the core of your body. You can build a direct connection with spiritual life force, the Light Consciousness that transfers higher knowledge into your human mind and at the cellular level.

Creative visualization and conscious intentions are the methods of communication between the higher mind of Spirit and the physical realm of matter. You live in a holographic universe where consciousness travels through photon particle-waves into infinite projections of potential realities. By harnessing the power of your holographic mind/right brain/3rd Eye, you can create visions of your preferred future outcome. When you are tuned into the subtle guidance of inner Soul Presence you begin to sense/feel/see what is resonant with your true nature. By following the 'call of your heart' you are feeding life force magnetism into creative pursuits that match your soul purpose and life plan.

1. Start a vision board of selected images, photos, intentions and affirmations that energize you! Select visuals that you respond to emotionally and physically, without thought. This is a clear sign they are an energetic match to your true nature and soul purpose.

2. As you tap into the power of the holographic mind, work with the Quantum Access™ meditation and visualize your intentioned reality. Place yourself in the future outcome of your visions, feeling alive with life force and inner heart magnetism. When you can show up and commit 100% to your Soul purpose, you are fully present in the NOW moment. When you are devoted to your soul purpose and destiny, the Universe will show up and support you!

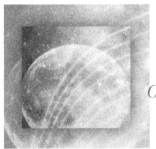

Chapter Six

THE SHADOW SELF

WE'VE HEARD OFTENTIMES from sages that the true path to enlightenment is the total acceptance of the shadow self. These wise beings encourage us to surrender into the "dark night of the Soul" in order to reach enlightenment! This process of Soul integration includes embracing all aspects of our being—both positive and negative. Yes, in order to become whole, healthy, complete beings, we need to face our shadow selves and compassionately accept and heal these lost fragments of consciousness.

In Debbie Ford's compelling book, *The Dark Side of the Light Chasers*, she discusses how our social mask is "the face we show the world. Unconcealing our shadow reveals our mask. We must look at this mask with love and compassion for there is great value in understanding what we hide behind." This healing process requires digging deep inside, observing and confronting our wounded human self, the part of our being that has suffered in the Time Matrix. It requires an offer of solace, gentle care, and a release from the painful shadow stored in cellular memory. This is not an easy or comfortable process but it's imperative to connect to ALL energy present within the human energy field so that we can piece ourselves back together again.

I would bet that most human beings believe they are good people and don't have a shadow self. This is testament to how much we are in denial of the dark nature of the Ego. As a society, we can no longer ignore the elephant in the room! Although we've learned how to split out and ignore the shadow self, it doesn't make it go away! Our personal blinders are not magical erasers that hide our dark side from view! The delusional mind is convinced it does, but the sad truth is that we're only fooling ourselves. Not only does the outer world mirror our patterns and programs back to us, but it reflects the hidden truth until we resolve it.

> "Everyone carries a shadow, and the less it is embodied in the individual's conscious life, the blacker and denser it is. At all counts, it forms an unconscious snag, thwarting our most well-meant intentions."
> • Carl G. Jung

Dealing with shadow consciousness has become a huge industry in our culture—we see increasing numbers of healers, psychiatrists, addiction rehab centers, marriage counselors, conflict resolution facilitators, divorce lawyers, financial debt consolidators, and the list goes on and on. This begs the question "why is humanity so ill?" What is causing the demise of the Human Spirit? Not only have I asked this question of myself, but I've also been faced with this question every time I start working with a new client. What seeds of separation could be causing such pain, suffering and dysfunction? The answers come when we begin to examine the shadow self.

Taking Back Our Lives

Why is shadow consciousness the root cause of separation—and how do we heal it?. After my walk-in experience, I was drowning in Darkness and could barely function. I was all alone, struggling with inner demons. I knew on some level that I had to get help, and that life as it existed was not acceptable. Due to enduring childhood Ritual Abuse, I was dealing with a fragmented mind in a fractured energy field.

In the end, it really comes down to territory. We need to take our human territory back and transform it into a Sacred vessel. We live in a parasitic world, controlled by a planetary program of parasitic consumerism. We also exist in a polarized system of positive and negative forces. For every positive action, there is an equal and compelling negative reaction. This polarized tension is alive in our own bodies, hearts and minds. It plays out in all areas of our lives, constantly sabotaging any progress with a downward spiral of negative counter-force. We cannot escape the very physics of our holographic reality just by denying that it exists.

"Growth is a detox process, as our weakest, darkest places are sucked up to the surface in order to be released..."

● Marianne Williamson

What is truly amazing about this paradox is that the very act of denial is causing deep internal separation the mind and physical energy. The very notion that we may be Dark or have a shadow self is both repelling and unacceptable to the righteous, grandiose Ego. But there is the catch—our personal Darkness *is*, in part, the denial of separation and the subsequent pain it creates. By ignoring our baser nature, the narcissism of the Ego and the complete lack of Soulful connection, we are operating in a world of emotional and Spiritual bankruptcy, which leads to egoic dominance, control and indulgence.

Eckhart Tolle so beautifully illuminates in *The Power of Now* the transformative effect of surrendering to '"what is" ... how it is not a passive act of failure, defeat or giving up, but an empowering act of acceptance. He says, "Surrender is the simple but profound wisdom of *yielding to* rather than *opposing* the flow of life ... the only place where you can experience the flow of life is the NOW." For it is in the Stillness of the Moment, the quiet, calm balance-point, that we can create the vacuum effect to draw Spirit within and be nourished. When the Ego is focused on a past memory or a future expectation, it is blocking the NOW and depriving us of the nourishment of Spirit. The shadow Ego is a by-product of Time! Only in the NOW Moment, where the Ego does not exist, can we experience Soul connection and the flow of Universal Abundance.

> "When we are alone and quiet, we are afraid that something will be whispered in our ear, and so we hate the silence and drug ourselves with social life."
>
> • Friedrich Nietzsche

The Identity Programs of Polarity

We are living in a world being pulled apart at the seams by the opposing forces of Light and Dark, and we need to resolve this polarity within our own human energy field. From the moment we enter this world at birth, we are pulled into the program of Duality. Depending on human DNA, place of birth, and family patterns, we adopt either the extreme egoic identity program of worthless insecurity, or the opposing identity of superior grandiosity.

Neither identity is healthy or balanced, but actually the human embodiment of positive or negative forces in our mental and emotional constructs and behavioral patterns. The healing process will balance the insecurity with authentic self-esteem, self-love and confidence, and balance the grandiosity with humility, empathy and compassion. Both extreme positions are balanced with Love!

A Quantum Leap Looms

When we discuss the nature of shadow, it embodies the absence of unconditional love. It is heavy, dense, oppressive and the absence of Light. It can range from painful emotions, vengeful judgments, psychic attacks, or energetic vampirism—all are examples of the absence of love and mutual receptivity. And since we all live in this world of Light and Dark, we all have acted within varying degrees of non-loving action (shadow). No one is exempt, no matter how much the Ego would like to delude us.

Yet Gregg Braden asserts that "the minimum number of people required to 'jumpstart' a change in consciousness is 1% of the population." This is sometimes termed the "Hundredth Monkey Effect", whereby new learned behavior will spread to other non-local communities through the morphogenetic field once a critical number of people adopting the behavior have been reached. New Age author, Ken Keyes Jr., further explored this theory in his book, *The Hundredth Monkey*, and illustrates how humanity is currently at the brink of a quantum leap in the collective consciousness

According to *The Mayan Code*, by Barbara Hand Clow, the "time cycles of the Mayan Calendar match important periods of evolutionary data banks in Earth and the Milky Way Galaxy". Clow believes we are "right in the middle of an overwhelming intellectual waking-up process."

The planetary alignment with the Galactic Center in 2012 altered the dynamics of polarity by introducing a neutralizing factor—the Zero Point Field of the Universe. We are entering this stage of human history with the profound knowledge and expertise of reaching a state of neutrality within the Void—the stillness between the anti-particle and particle fields of physical matter. Within the sacred geometry of Singularity, we are able to not only balance and neutralize human polarity but we can begin the process of transforming DNA by transmuting shadow with Love.

This process has escalated within recent months and years as more and more Souls awaken to the truth about human enslavement and genetic manipulation. This includes the insertion of genetic implants that code humanity to feed on emotionally charged energy instead of Universal Light. This genetic corruption has destroyed all sense of evolutionary potential and has locked the human race in a downward spiral of co-dependency, addiction, death and disconnection.

Confronting & Resolving Distortion

Humanity is being fueled by charged emotional energy and craves intense drama. Despite the fact that human conflict is extremely unpleasant and stressful, we feel drawn into the sordid mess to consume on negative emotions. Betrayed by our own inclinations, we cannot resist being pulled in and engaged in the battle with negative shadow forces.

Our primitive nature is coded to seek charged emotions instead of being fed by the natural stillness of the Universe. We are out of sync with the rhythm and flow of nature.

"Integrity is the absence of contradiction between what we know, what we profess and what we do."

• Nathanial Branden

Down through the ages, Karmic patterning repeats and builds upon itself. With focused research, we can observe and identify specific conflicts in our lives and trace the root cause to early childhood or parallel/past-livesr. This reveals the string of events leading up to the current imbalance, which alerts our awareness to remove the entire history of karmic patterning from our energy fields. In this manner, we can confront , resolve and remove the ancestral lineage of distorted shadow patterning from our consciousness and human energy field. The key is to find and remove the root so that the entire network collapses and releases.

Not only does the shadow program collapse, but all consciousness and DNA codes stored in the human energy field that were linked to that pattern will clear out as well. When we finally have resolved and cleared all karmic charge and the shadow patterning related to the root, we then witness the final collapse of the original timeline from the Human Energy Field. It literally drops out of our aura and sets us free!

So we must find the core root and more often than not it resides in early childhood or past-life trauma. This gets tricky for we need to locate the original source of shadow violation, which may even be in another timeline. Quantum Access™ opens the door to all timelines in the multi-dimensional Unified Field. While spinning in the timeless Quantum Vortex, we can trace a symptom, condition or distorted pattern and locate the root to clear out the entire network throughout all time. This healing process is profoundly effective in liberating our lives of stubborn, deeply engrained shadow programming.

What to Expect

As we begin the healing steps to clear all karmic timelines, we "awaken" to how much shadow is embedded and stored in our cells and chakras. It can feel overwhelming! Not only has the trauma been stored, but also the dark presence of violation. This is why we may feel haunted by suffocating fears, deeply wounded emotions, a fragmented mind and perhaps diseased body, but we are unable to pinpoint the cause. The energetic trauma of violation and persecution from other timelines is still charged and alive in the energy field. Doctors cannot find any reason; there's no evidence for trauma, fear or obsession. How often do we hear stories of very successful, affluent people in happy marriages, with healthy children, who commit suicide? Considering this from the surface level, it doesn't make sense! But the shadow is real and wielding enormous impact on the quality of life.

Facing and healing the shadow self and shadow consciousness is a significant step in becoming whole again! We cannot skip this step and then expect to ascend in vibration to reach apotheosis. For it is our personal shadow that keeps us stuck in victim consciousness and trapped in the parasitic hologram. I had an irrational fear of being known and visible in public as a healer or teacher. It took years before I could even place my photo on my business materials and website. I traced my phobia back to past-lives cut short by persecution and murder. This personal trauma was deep inside, holding me frozen in fear of more persecution. It became an energetic doorway into my human energy field for more violation to occur. This is why it is so important that we heal all past-life trauma and deep wounds, so that we can clear and remove all access points or portals to the externalworld/astral plane.

We must become aware that shadow exists in myriad forms of Darkness, and we need to recognize where it is active within our own energy, in our behavior, and in our daily lives. We are Spiritual warriors of the Light! We must face how shadow manipulates, seduces and destroys our connection to Soul Precense and the abundant Universe. It is divisive in nature and hell-bent on dominating our will and splitting us apart. The motto of Darkness is "divide and conquer"! As I became more aware of how polarity works, and how shadow tricks and invades our energy field, I went on hyper-alert … not only in myself but also with my clients. The more I uncovered, the more I realized how most of us are being overly influenced by outside Dark forces of psychic attacks, feeder lines, parasitic astral entities, bacterial and viral invasions, spells and curses, patterns from the family of origin, corrupted reptilian hyrbrid genetics, religious persecution, witchcraft, OK … you get the drift.

All of these examples are divisive forms of shadow consciousness—all invisible to the human eye and yet wreaking havoc in our lives. To be honest with you, I wouldn't have believed it existed either until I saw it for myself. But we don't have to wait until our clairvoyance is fully operational, just feel how painful Darkness has affected our lives. I bet you can come up with a whole list of examples when you have felt disconnected, stuck, haunted, spied on, cursed or insecure. We don't have to be psychic to know something's messing with us!

Defenses Against the Shadow

As children, we developed ways to escape the pain of shadow, usually creating methods of splitting out of our bodies and floating in the ethers to feel hidden and safe. Unfortunately these coping mechanisms only accomplish temporary relief for the mind and emotions, but cannot prevent the violation of Darkness in our human energy fields. As children, we established escapist patterns or coping mechanism that fragmented the mind and fractured the human Bio-Energetics. We're seeing more and more evidence of this pattern showing up in medical conditions such as ADHD, OCD, autism, schizophrenia, post-traumatic syndrome, compulsive eating, delusion and emotional immaturity. By the time we become adults, we've developed a deeply engrained behavioral pattern to split out under any stressful situation. No wonder we're walking around like zombies, ungrounded and confused.

> "What! Must I hold a candle to my shames?"
> • William Shakespeare

Now I recognize this is not a popular topic, and in the earlier years of my awakening, I shied away from it myself. I was determined to only focus on love and light! Well I could stay in denial only for so long... for guess what kept coming up—all forms of shadow consciousness. We don't realize how easily the mind and emotions can be influenced by outside forces. Meanwhile, if the human self is splitting out, then we are more at risk for outside manipulation.

Transforming the Darkness

I have found shadow can influence and invade our relationships, our addictive cravings, mental anguish, OCD obsessions, our emotional rage and paranoia. It shows up in extreme reactions to commonplace events! It manifests as psychic spying and repeated appearances in our minds of disturbing people from our past. We need to pay attention and recognize that the marjority of our daily thoughts, emotional reactions or behavior do not originate from our authentic self. We need to hunt down Darkness and transform it!

The path to healing shadow lies within us, for we can no longer avoid the pain, the suffering and the haunting Darkness we encounter in our daily lives. It is real and can be healed. We must look for patterns of separation, the extreme reactions, mind-control programs, addictions, any haunting presence around the body, in the mind, and in the home. We need to watch for disturbances in our intimate relationships, where we are closing our hearts, pushing others away with rage, jealousy, attacks, neediness or infidelity. These are examples of shadow infiltration.

In order to transform ourselves into Divine Humans, we need to dig deep, investigate and uncover all areas of distortions and irregularities within ourselves. Our original Soul nature is a pure reflection of Universal Love. So if Love is our true essence, than the absence of Love is Darkness. Keep it simple, and apply healing touch to all energy present that is void of Love. With this approach, we begin the healing process of transforming ourselves from broken, separated humans into whole, Divine beings. By setting this intent, we initiate the healing process of "internal house-cleaning."

A Powerful Choice

Usually we need to wait for karmic life events to trigger opportunities in our daily lives for healing and resolution. These karmic triggers can materialize such as bank snafus, lost checks, relationship betrayals, accidents, broken electronics, sexual dysfunction, or physical pain and illness. Since most of human reality is controlled by the Ego will, all karmic triggers are processed through our physical existence.

I finally reached a point in my healing where I said, "Enough is enough." I was done with triggering karma in my physical life. I was ready to raise it up to the Soul level and process all shifts in consciousness in the higher realms. In this manner, we can elevate the conduit for learning and Spiritual growth to flow in from higher wisdom, like "aha moments" of awareness. It requires surrendering Ego control over the physical life, and "yielding" to the Soul all lessons and life decisions.

In the groundbreaking book, *A New Earth*, Eckhart Tolle discusses how the Ego treats the present moment as the enemy. He says that "Time, past and future, is what the ego lives on ... and time is in your mind. The elimination of time from your consciousness is the elimination of ego. It is the only true spiritual practice." By meditating within the Quantum Vortex, we are able to quiet the mind, step out of time and embrace the NOW, create the stillness of balance, dissolve ego resistance, and breathe Divine Love into our hearts.

If Darkness is the absence of Love, then the most effective tonic to use in healing internal shadow is self-love. The more love we flow into our deepest wounds and darkest emotions, the quicker we are able to clear and raise our vibration, thus elevating the process of spiritual growth from the realm of physical mishaps or triggers. This process gradually transforms us into a powerful, healthy Divine Human experiencing "heaven on earth." This is our destiny and our purpose!

No longer dependent on a pre-destined karmic blueprint, we become free to create what heart magnetism. As we re-connect to Universal abundance, we move away from the empty VOID, and into the Quantum Field of unlimited potential.

Envision a world reality where all that exists is available within the grand force field we live in. We can embrace the vastness of the Quantum Field of all possibilities as our new playground. We are now living in a "blank canvas" awaiting the first brush stroke of our brilliance. As the hidden artist crawls out of the emptiness and begins to create with boldness, we must still heal and nurture the bruised and battered human being that has lost its bearings.

In summary, being trapped in a negative karmic cycle has fostered the powerful domination of the Ego identity and the subsequent rise of shadow consciousness in the mind/heart/body. The healing path leads to the "dark night of the Soul," as we dissolve Ego resistance, fill our hearts with love, regain control of our lives, and open to the flow and rhythm of the abundant Universe.

Healing Exercise

Karmic Resolution: Living as the Observer, you begin to flush out all hidden unconscious programs, scripts and patterns that are running in the background of your daily life. At first the Ego may recoil in denial and blame, incapable of acknowledging any responsibility for its existence. This is the tipping point of your healing process – do you sink back into unconscious behavior or do you accept the imbalances and initiate your personal healing transformation?

1. Create a sacred space for healing, activate Quantum Access™ … move into the Meditative state, focus on the discordant behavior pattern, belief, or blockage and allow yourself to feel how this energy impacts the quality of your life.
2. Ask your Higher Self to show you the full story – "why is it present, what is it teaching me, what is the gift/life lesson of wisdom I am receiving?"
3. As you analyze the energetic pattern without judgment, you

can take ownership of the karmic history and start to resolve all remaining issues involved to close the cycle.

When you are willing to accept and integrate the karmic wisdom, you can use the Quantum Vortex to dissolve all polarized charge around the pattern...neutralizing the energetic shadow to release from the human energy field. By bringing hidden unconscious patterns into the Light, you have the ability to reclaim lost or stuck power, raise your vibration and regain inner balance in your central core.

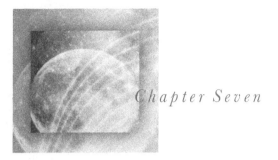

Chapter Seven

THE ENSLAVEMENT OF HUMANITY

THERE WAS A time when our ancestors lived in freedom and sovereignty, experiencing the totality of their Soul gifts and knowledge, as well as the abundance inherent to all living creatures. We still carry within our human DNA the hidden memories of those sweet times past, and can begin to activate and accelerate the return to such a world reality again. It's been a long road getting here, but the journey has been enlightening to say the least. At this point, I'm sure many of you are asking: *How did we get here in the first place? Why are so many still asleep? Why are most people not aware of the current conditions of human enslavement, and how do we wake up the world around us?*

These are questions I ask myself during quiet hours of reflection, when I struggle to envision how the world can turn around in time. But it is in these moments of seeking that I find the crystal-clear truth of how we got here and why, and how we can liberate ourselves from entrapment and enter into freedom.

A Collective Amnesia

The global collective mind has amnesia, being under the spell of genetic manipulation and a planetary artificial computer simulation. It is as if we are sleep-walking through our lives, not recognizing that some external force is directing our thoughts, feelings and urges.

> "The important thing is to be able at any moment to sacrifice what we are for what we could become."
>
> • Charles Dubois

According to renowned medium and best-selling author James Van Praagh, "When people shed their physical bodies at death, their spiritual selves see life from a whole new perspective. It's as if they had Lasik surgery. They can finally take off their glasses and see everything more clearly. Spirits understand why certain situations had to happen. They are able to recognize the value of others, even their enemies, and what they had to learn from them. They also realize how they could have skipped certain mistakes by not letting their egos get in the way."

The program of entrapment streams through the ego mind, powerful programming of separation which has been implanted into the reptilian brain stem, spinal column and biological nervous system. Everywhere I searched, I found that human DNA has been corrupted with divisive codes and templates that prevent connection to our Spiritual selves. This is why we cannot integrate our fertile, vibrant spiritual existence within our earth-bound reality.

Since we have amnesia, we are not even aware of what freedoms we have lost. When I peer into the Master Receptor Cell of the human race, I find corrupted codes designed to eliminate the Spiritual quotient of human beings. This leaves humanity living within a shell of physical biology without the engine to drive it.

Split from Our Divine Soul

Centuries past, as the hybridized human began to populate, an ever-increasing split occurred between the physical self and the Soul presence. This began to create an entirely new alternate personality or Ego identity. Over time, this new personality grew into the commanding consciousness of the human will and could be manipulated by the invader race. They achieved this by stimulating the nervous system and brain stem with inserted scalar field activity to impose further conditions like mind-control programming.

All thoughts, feelings and behavioral impulses were being fed from a hidden external source, with the intent to generate a certain biosphere of energized material to distract and dominate human consciousness.

Once the polarized Matrix was established, the experiment become the norm, and an underlying system of Duality developed that created a continuing feast of negatively charged energy. It became an opposing force field of positive and negative charge that wrapped around the planet and invaded our biological environment and mental activity. We see this polarized web at work in the endless pursuit of material acquisition and the cycle of "victim-persecution" that draws us in and keeps us trapped.

In a way, it's like being held prisoner in a jail, where we can envision freedom and our full potential, but we cannot break free of the prison walls holding us in. These walls are energetic membranes, or frequency fences, of coded consciousness inserted into our minds, our hearts, within the cellular makeup, and around our bodies to prevent any connection to Source Creator or our Divine Soul. Our energetic prison is keeping us living in a very limited, fearful state of entrapment.

Cut Off from Joy & Abundance

We see examples of enslavement within our personal existence, in the very nature of how we relate to each other and to planet

Earth. We see the seeds of corruption alive and well within the dysfunctional relationship model of co-dependency and boundary race wars between countries. Wherever we are feeling others have more than us, this is an example of the deprivation consciousness which limits our access to universal abundance. We call this the "Have-Have Not's" program of separation. The power elite have access to wealth and prosperity, and those who are in the energetic prison are cut off from all access.

> "That which we do not bring to consciousness appears in our lives as fate."
> • Carl G. Jung

I could literally see and feel the "line of demarcation" barrier in front of my body preventing me from crossing over and accessing what I needed. It was heart-wrenching not being able to provide for my needs. I was entangled within this prison mentality and fear-based survival program. It affected all areas of my life and invaded my thoughts and feelings on a continual basis. I could not find rest or reprieve anywhere from this prison, except in quiet meditation. Without any real connection to Spirit in my earthly reality,

I eventually sought spiritual nourishment in the astral plane. I had to split out of my biological vessel in order to connect to Spiritual energy. I began to live the majority of my waking hours split out of my body, no longer grounded into my earthly life. This led to other problems and my energy field became a hosting ground for energy vampirism. So neither option really worked.

It wasn't until I mastered using the Quantum Vortex, that I could break free of my energetic prison and experience freedom again. As the membranes of time thinned and began to open, I was able to travel far and wide in the astral realm and discover the true nature of humanity. What a joy it was to see our heritage and how free we used to be. I vowed I would live this way again!

Breaking Free with Meditation

Since we have been living within the karmic trap of Duality and separation from Spirit, we have not been able to access our superconscious mind, or intuitive awareness. The Ego intercepts and blocks the mind's natural connection to higher knowing, our access to the dynamic energetic lattice of Universal Intelligence. We operate liked trained robots, allowing the Ego mind to make decisions and direct our life. This is a tough pattern to break, and most people find it difficult to know what resonates with Soul truth or not. We have been living split and separated from our Higher Knowing all these incarnations, and we will need to relearn how to trust and follow the Soul guidance.

As we integrate the body, mind, emotions and Spirit into more holistic union, we strengthen our ability to feel and sense the vibration of all things. The highest frequency of joy and Love occurs when the Soul and the Human Self have come together in union. The lowest frequency of energy is the absence of Love and deep Soul disconnection.

The Quantum Vortex is the most effective tool we have to break free of Ego control. As we breathe into the inner stillness and quiet the mental chatter, we eliminate Ego resistance. For it is in the quiet Still-Point field that Spirit awakens in our hearts and beings! The neutralized, non-polarized state of stillness creates a vacuum effect that draws Spirit into our conscious awareness. When the Ego mind is barking out orders, criticisms, fears or worries, we are splitting into separation from our Spiritual energy. In order to ascend we need to adopt a regular meditation practice, to awaken the cellular memory of your human heritage and energetic chalice for Spiritual union.

The Harmful Ego Self

The Ego self is dominated and controlled by a global Mind Matrix of streaming commands, beliefs, fears, and diminishing consciousness. Since the "Fall of Man," the collective mind continues to proliferate the shadow program.

If you think about it—the Ego is insatiable, always feeling alone, craving pleasure and immediate gratification. We can never fully satisfy it, for the Ego always wants more!

This constant hunger drives the mental focus outwards to feed on external sources. In the pursuit of fulfillment, the Ego personality continually creates more inner separation. This is the "do loop" of human consumerism. The Big Lie perpetuated throughout planetary consciousness is that acquisition will make us happy! In reality, it will keep us trapped in perpetual separation from our Souls. When we confront this lie within our own mind, the Ego recoils—just try it! I can hear my Ego screaming, "Don't take consumerism away from me! I will starve!!"

> "It is in the nature of things to be drawn to the very experiences that will spoil our innocence, transform our lives, and give us necessary complexity and depth."
> • Thomas Moore

That, my friends, is the program inserted in our minds to destroy our power, our Spirit, and our innate ability to create and manifest. We must break free in order to evolve and ascend into becoming Divine Humans. Once we understand that the Ego is sabotaging our dreams and invading our inner harmony, then we can begin to distance ourselves and detach from its grasp. This requires paying attention to all the voices running in the background, in the subconscious mind as well, so that we can move into alignment with the subtle, peaceful, loving inner voice of the Soul. We need to embrace our Inner Wiser Self and disengage from our harmful Ego self.

This can be done in meditation, with an energy healer, with a Spiritual therapist, or with friends who understand this healing process and can provide a sounding board as witnesses to the debilitating patterns of the corrupted Ego. We cannot do this alone, for the Ego will trick us. We need loving supportive feedback when the program is still controlling our thoughts, feelings or behavior. It's time to get real with each other, and compassionately be present with honesty and integrity as we all move through the Ascension Process.

Disengaging from Corruption

The Mind Matrix appears energetically like an oppressive black web plugged into our primal reptilian brain stem, spine and chakras. We need to disengage from the entire corrupted system in order to activate our Divine lineage. As we break each egoic pattern and clear out more karmic debt, we raise our energy frequency and weaken the hold the dark web has on us. As we breathe crystallized Light into the cells, we are strengthening our energetic container and activating the Light Body to merge with Soul Presence. All of these steps contribute to feeling more whole and empowered, breaking free from the Time Matrix and disentangling from the web of Duality.

> "Transformation does not start with some one else changing you; transformation is an inner self reworking of what you are now to what you will be."
>
> • Byron Pulsifer

It is imperative that we receptive beings again. For without this skill, we cannot receive the abundance of the Universe. Due to the interfering Ego, we have been living separated and cut off from Spiritual energy ... hardening into closed-off shells of emptiness. Our bodies have become dense, hard-edged and rigid. Our wounded hearts have become guarded, defensive and yearning for Love. Our minds have become a breeding ground for negative criticism, anger and vengeful reactions.

In order to reverse the damage, we need to disentangle out of the Dark web of control, distance ourselves from the insidious insatiable Ego mind, and rebuild our energetic container. As we transform ourselves from the inside out, we can begin to train our body intelligence to soften, open and receive the sustenance of Universal nourishment. We switch the flow of energy from outgoiong, to incoming into the chakra pillar. In this way, we retrain our physical energy to let down the guarded shields—we build auric shields in place to protect us—and we can slowly open our receptors sites to be fed the manna from heaven.

How many of us have seen our dreams and desires vanquished by invading forces in the form of greed, jealousy, betrayal and deceit? How much of our lives have been thwarted due to the polarized shadow forces invading our mind and body? We ask ourselves why we haven't found our Divine Lover, our life's work, our Soul purpose? These are the costs we've paid.

The planetary Matrix hologram has prevented our Soul from fulfilling our destiny, as we suffer endlessly from the loss of freedom. No Soul should be living in pain, lack or neglect. It is not the Law of the Universe. Now is the time to focus our mind with the intent to break free and reunite with our Divine Spirit.

In summary, the global collective mind has been under a spell of amnesia and genetic reengineering, which has separated humanity from Spiritual energy and the vast Universal abundance. Meditation in the Quantum Vortex provides the sacred key we need to unlock the prison walls of the 3D Time Matrix and the web of darkness.

Healing Exercise

Power of Imagination: Acting as the 'Observer' in life, you start to notice the internal dialogue occurring between your human self and the higher self. This may include a complex array of topics ranging from mundane chores you need to do or the idiosyncrasies of the people around you…to the many hidden hopes, dreams, and aspirations you desire to achieve in life. The key to enlightenment is to unlock these precious nuggets of Soul truth that slide into your awareness as you filter through the enormous tidal wave of distraction, distortions, illusions, disappointments, self-sabotage, anger and blame.

Once you begin to understand that you really are not your 'mind', but a vital, spiritual essence breathing life into a complex network of biological parts and circuits that form your human reality. Your life force is the embodiment of eternal Source, and you have the ability to break free of the prison of 3D density and transform your human limitations into what dreams are made of.

Now begin to add to your healing journal all the ways your higher self is communicating to you – be it in the dream state, in imagination, in sharing your inner hopes, listing what makes you feel happy, energized, and amped with excitement. This provides valuable insight into the Soul essence waiting to manifest in your life.

In this process you will gain more awareness of the deep, inner spiritual wealth rising up to the surface to come alive and be expressed in the world. It is the negative thoughts, emotions and self-defeating patterns of behavior that interfere with our natural Soul gifts blossoming inside. When we pay attention to our hopes and dreams of becoming a divine human…we can begin to align with our Soul's greater plan and feed it our life force.

For example, my higher self communicates valuable insights about the current condition of my energy with 'house' dreams. How the house appears in my dreams mirrors my personal situation. If the house is missing walls or a ceiling, I am being guided to integrate a vital piece of my infrastructure. If my house is being invaded, I need to strengthen my energetic shields and clear out violation. If my house is too small, I need to expand and open up to more of my inner power and abundance. I have learned so much valuable information from my higher self in a variety of 'house' dreams for the past 20 years. Pay attention and observe how your Soul is guiding you!

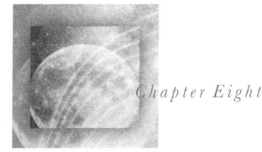

Chapter Eight

VICTIM CONSCIOUSNESS

WE ARE AT a point in timey where humanity can rise out of the malaise of victim-consciousness. More and more people are awakening to the truth! If you look around, you will see signs of a new awareness of global injustices and the call for change. This will increase as our minds shift in the sands of evolutionary advancement.

Our past-life memory is stored in the Akashic Records in the superconscious mind or timeless mind. Our current life memory is stored in the 3rd- dimensional human mind—in memory banks like a computer database. Not only is the imprint of every event stored in memory banks, but also the mental perspective, the emotional feelings, and the physical reactions.

Dr. Fred Alan Wolf, a theoretical physicist, studied Quantum Physics and its relationship to consciousness. He says that matter is how Spirit appears in the physical Universe, and how matter appears depends on our mind's choices. In other words, we create our current reality by the continual choices that we make. Our "Unified Field" translates into a human hologram where our inner condition is interwoven with the materialization of our physical lives.

This substantiates how incredibly powerful the mind is in determining the actual form our lives take. This also points to how dangerous it can be if our subconscious minds are being programmed, without our permission or knowledge, with divisive patterning, fears and distortions.

A Downward Spiral

It has become clear from many years doing Quantum Healing, that from the onset of human birth we get plugged into the 3D Time Matrix programming, which is stored in the mind's memory banks. This programming begins to form into a false ego-identity, an alternate personality that controls our lives, and asserts its will in opposition to our Spiritual growth. The Ego sees itself as separate from Spirit as well as being separate in the Universe. Due to the very nature of setting itself apart, the Ego begins to feel alone and vulnerable, no longer loved and supported by a benevolent Universe. This sets the stage for the endless cycle of opposing forces of positive/negative energy to play out in the Ego's imagined reality. Thus, we become entrapped in the deeply engrained "Victim-Persecution" program, the karmic loop of human Duality.

"The biggest disease today is not leprosy or tuberculosis, but rather the feeling of being unwanted, uncared for and deserted by everybody."

• Mother Teresa

Since the Ego exists as a separate entity from its surrounding world, it begins to experience more isolation, emptiness, loneliness and paranoia – experiencing the "me against the world" mentality. Disconnection from the abundant Universe breeds a sense of lack and deprivation, living a life of struggle and strife.

This creates a reality of feeling deprived, punished and denied life support, and so the Victim Identity begins. When we no longer feel fed, nurtured or supported in life, this erodes healthy self-esteem and confidence. Our sense of self dissolves into a disturbing sensation that something is missing inside us—leaving us feeling "less than," insecure, broken, shameful and/or bad.

Eventually the Victim Identity is driven to seek whatever it can attain from the external world to fill the empty hole inside. We begin to go outside ourselves to feed on others' energy, and become trapped in the co-dependent model of relationship. Of course, external dependencies erode all sense of wholeness, creating an underlying belief that we need to merge with another human being to complete us.

This destructive programming triggers a downward spiral into deeper and darker emotions, building into a powerful quagmire of negatively charged toxic emotional energy! It gets stuck looping in the mind and pulsing in the sensory body. Eventually the stored toxins degrade physical health and manifest in illness and disease. Author Eckhart Tolle (*Power of Now, The New Earth*) says that when you become ill, "if you complain, feel self-pity, or resent being ill, your ego becomes stronger ... especially if you make the illness part of your conceptual identity." How often have you heard someone claim with pride, like a badge of honor, that they are Victims of such and such a disease?

Depleted & Searching

We are functioning like cars running on empty, depleted and drained of our natural fuel – the energy of Creation. As you know, all of life is a form of energy. And so the Ego is on a mission to seek, find and consume energy anywhere it can access it. We've lost our lifeline to the abundant Universe, so we are doing our best to survive in separation. The two most powerful sources of energy that we seek are Love and Money! It is a battle to acquire as much Love and Money as we can consume. We become obsessed in pursuing Love in our co-dependent relationships, and acquiring money to feed our material consumerism. But it's never enough. We still feel empty inside! Due to victim-consciousness, we feel disconnected from our personal power, fending for ourselves in a chaotic world. We do not feel supported or cared for by an abundant Universe. We're stuck in a vicious cycle of seeking fulfillment from outside sources of energy, and then resenting the partner, the job or family we are dependent on. It's a crushing system and set up to keep us trapped in our dependencies.

Consequences of a Victim Mentality

> "Our deepest fear is not that we are inadequate. Our deepest fear is that we are powerful beyond measure. It is our light, not our darkness, that most frightens us."
> • Marianne Williamson

If you take a look around you there are infinite examples of how humanity has fallen prey to the insidious program of victim-consciousness. We are currently witnessing in our global economy the karmic payback of corporate greed—that "me against the world" mentality in our financial services and banking system. This type of greed for money and power has no moral sense of consequence to the customer. Not only does the victim's fear of lack motivate greed into hoarding, but breeds an underlying sense of anxiety and 'survival fear'.

Another example of moral corruption is evident in Wall Street's gambling on the housing market, gaming the system and then betting against it. This defies the Universal Law of Compensation. Taking without giving back goes against the rhythm of nature and the ebb and flow of an equal energy exchange.

There is nothing substantiating the income earned, since it is capitalizing on other people's hard work without any investment of energy. The public is beginning to realize that without a balanced exchange, capitalism has degraded into a corrupted usury system and cannot sustain itself. It is out of balance with the rhythms of nature and is currently beginning to collapse like a house of cards.

We cannot sustain a healthy society when the mind has been corrupted with victim-consciousness. When we doubt our personal abundance, we are no longer capable of owning our full potential as manifesters! According to Quantum Mechanics, all our thoughts and feelings are recorded into the stream of consciousness that creates our human reality. When we operate in victim consciousness, we are projecting a world reality of scarcity and sabotaging our personal abundance

Learning to Source Divine Energy

Once I realized how harmful this behavior was to my personal safety and financial security, I became much more aware and vigilant in supplying my own life force. I began meditating regularly to fill with spiritual Energy inside. With regular practice, my ability to source my own life with the fuel of the Universe, which is Love Energy, grew and multiplied. I recognized that Divine Light was streaming into my heart on a regular basis and had expanded and filled my Inner Core with Love. I had never experienced such Joy and felt so much Love within me. It grew in intensity and power with continual meditation in the Quantum Vortex. I learned how to fill my inner emptiness with an endless stream of Love Energy, and noticed that I wasn't splitting out of my body like before. I followed the mantra my guides gave me: "Do not go outside myself for anything!" I repeated this over and over, drilling it

> "Someone who does not know how to receive love will, of course, end up feeling unloved."
> • Marianne Williamson

into my subconscious mind, so I could break the harmful pattern of victim dependency and scarcity struggle. I began to rebuild my human energy field from all the past fragmenting. My Inner Chakra Pillar had become my new home, a haven of safety and source nourishment.

Confronting the Ego

As I set my intention to source my own life force, an awakening occurred—I was able to claim my personal Soul Sovereignty. I set about letting go of all co-dependent relationships and owning my personal responsibility to provide for myself. This triggered egoic fear and resistance to "stand on my own." I had to face and heal all my human anxiety around feeling less than, insecure, self-doubt and neediness. This rose to the surface in the form of debilitating victim-consciousness and had to go!

Due to lifetimes of repeated patterns of victimization, I dicovered the Ego's distrust of self and Soul and any ability to provide fundamental needs. The Ego does not believe it can successfully survive as an independent being. This is all rooted in victim-consciousness. Since my mind did not believe I could provide, I therefore resisted claiming responsibility for myself. I gave away my personal power to my family, my partners, my friends, my teachers, the Ascended Masters. Since I didn't trust myself, I turned to others to provide for me. My Inner Core had become Void of all power.

Magnetizing Our Core

As we proclaim to the Universe our Soul Sovereignty, we begin to transform the inner empty Void-space to become the vacuum of power. In quantum mechanics, within the Zero-Point Field exists a vacuum state of empty space and stillness. It is a null-zone, void of gravity. When we meditate within the zero point of the Quantum Vortex and activate the Universal Harmonic

Tones, or sacred geometry of *phi* (the golden ratio of Order and Divine proportion), we begin to create within our Chakra Pillar a vacuum state that will draw in what we need.

We can replace the old state of emptiness to become a sacred space for union and wholeness. By guiding the human consciousness through the steps to release Victim Identity and embrace Soul Identity, we can initiate the profound process of activating authentic Soul Union.

The key is to recognize the voice and feelings of the victim inside, and to heal the wound. Then we disengage from the energetic pattern—and let it go. Next, we need to turn within and fill up inside with unconditional love, breathing Soul Presence into the Chakra Pillar ... pooling in the heart center. We need to concentrate on replacing the old habit of reaching outside to consume, and instead remain inside our body ... staying present, not splitting out.

Life as Powerful Sovereign Beings

> "We have no more right to consume happiness without producing it than to consume wealth without producing it."
>
> • George Bernard Shaw

By living in the Core of our bodies, we begin to get more grounded, rooted in the earthly realm. This enables the kundalini life force to increase and grow as a wellspring within, igniting an internal engine of magnetism. When we eliminate the energetic leaks and drains, and build inner reserves of Spiritual life force, we are essentially creating a powerful force field of magnetic attraction. Not only does this provide an endless source of physical energy, but it also generates a compelling magnetic power to manifest in the material world. It is not a mental exercise to manifest! It is visceral and invigorating! The more present we are in our heart center, the more magnetic power we have to draw in what we need from the abundant Universe.

The human holographic reality begins to transform into a benevolent Universe of endless Love and nourishment. By taking the lead to source our own life force as powerful Sovereign Beings, we leave behind the painful separation of victim consciousness and embrace the endless supply of Universal Love. By feeding our human energy field a continual stream of Love Energy, we activate the heart magnetics to attract loving relationships and financial support.

By correcting the intention of our thoughts, choices and desires, we can transform the molecular patterning that creates our human experience. The quantum notion of discontinuity and the illusion of time and space also provide a transformational opportunity. When life doesn't occur in a linear fashion in time, then we can transcend the past in one moment. By spinning within the timeless Quantum Vortex, we can jump into a totally spontaneous newly formed present, released from past conditioning ... ready to experience life with new freshness, hope and purpose.

In summary, the debilitating "victim-persecutor" pattern prevents human evolution, impairs creative manifestation, and sabotages prosperity and well-being. Victim consciousness is the most effective shadow-programming to destroy human potential and eliminate Love and compassion in our lives.

Healing Exercise

Observation: In order to break free of the enslavement of the Time Matrix, you must nuetralize polarized opposition, eliminate the Karmic Incarnational trap and subsequent Victim-Persecutor program. As long as you swing back and forth within the identities of feeling Victimized or enraged Persecutor, you will continue to sink into the cloying, dark web of Duality.

Disallow the Ego to indulge in feelings of "being wronged" or obsessive needs to balance the imagined offense with "getting back" at the offender. This can only happen when you take responsibility for all that occurs in your reality, knowing it is reflecting back to you where you are still polarized and out-of-balance.

When you start to see your life as mirror reflections of your inner condition, you can own it, and start to transform it. This en gages a new inner dialogue that analyzes life events with the intent to investigate thoroughly all aspects of the hidden subconscious self. Your approach to life is now focused on disclosing clues and insights to where youe are still polarized.

1. Put on your Investigator's cap...you are now the private detector sleuthing out all polarized Victim-Persecutor programs enslaving you in the Karmic Cycle of Duality.

2. Whenever you become aware of feeling victimized or seeking revenge...proclaim "STOP" in your mind to the shadow ego! Do not give it your power, your attention or your life force!

3. Claim your inner power to shift the reality into a new energy of neutral, detached acceptance—as an opportunity to gain more wisdom, and hold your balanced Still Point! Do not allow any energy to pull you into the opposing forces of Duality!

Reinforce your commitment to live outside of the dark web of the Time Matrix, to break free and live as a Sovereign Being!

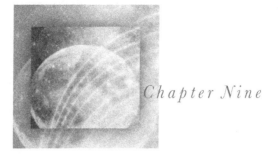

Chapter Nine

A CONTAINER OF LIGHT

IF WE TRAVEL back in time to the original human blueprint and the birth of a new civilization, we see the Original Human Being created in the image of God/ Goddess. It was a beautiful act of Love, this creation of Spirit in physical form. These original humans were placed within a lush, resplendent ecosystem, often referred to as the Garden of Eden. The original humans were nourished by Divine Energy and communicated telepathically. They were the perfect embodiment of Sacred Union, a balanced unified blend of masculine and feminine energy. These humans were God/Goddess realized, and they lived in perfect harmony in the Universal Field of ONE.

The original human Souls are our ancestors, and we carry the cellular memory of Sacred Union in our genetic blueprint. Our goal within this Ascension Plan is to come full circle and realize the full potential of the original human tribe. We need to clear out the genetic corruption, repltilian hybrid lineage and any distortions that prevent the activation of the 12-strand DNA, in order to activate the full capacity of our Divine Human ancestral lineage.

As we go back in time to the seed of corruption, we trace back to Mitochondrial Eve, the matriarchal ancestor from Africa who is linked to all humans living today. When spinning within the timeless Quantum Vortex, we can clear out the corrupted codes passed down generationally from Mitochondrial Eve and repair the damaged DNA. Not only do we need to clear out genetic implants and repair the human energy field, but we also need to rehabilitate the damaged human Spirit from the trauma and wounding of separation. As we move through the steps to rebuild and rebirth our Divine Human Energy Field, we are creating a "container" for Sacred Union.

Healing Our Heart Centers

The human heart center acts as the main hub of life force, similar to Grand Central Station—the heart center being the central conduit of energy throughout the entire auric field. Our heart center is the bridge that connects the human self to the Soul aspect in union and harmony, acting as the communication center for our Soul's desires, passion and inspiration. How many times have we been torn between the Ego's desires in the mind opposing the Soul's wishes in the heart? The heart-brain is the Soul's source of communication and guidance. Our challenge as human beings is learning how to pause, become still and listen, to follow the intuition and yearnings of the heart ... knowing that we are receiving Divine guidance.

If the heart is wounded from early childhood trauma, abuse and disconnection, it is challenging to feel anything, let alone Soulful guidance. From years of pain and suffering, our hearts have become guarded, closed up and tuned out! We figure it's better not to feel anything at all, than open the heart to feel immense pain again.

Unfortunately, this stance keeps us locked in isolation, and the heart center will never mend. As we begin the process of healing, we need to clear the genetic distortion and rehabilitate and rebirth the inner wounded child, in order to successfully repair and renew a healthy, happy heart.

By investing time and self-care into this healing process, we are liberating our human selves from the debilitating karmic destiny of cyclic reincarnation, from the prison of the Time Matrix, and from the original wound of separation. In this way, the human Spirit can recover, and regenerate with healthy selfesteem and confidence derived from Soul Presence, not from the false illusion of Ego grandiosity. A healthy heart is open, receptive and intuitive in nature. As we heal and mend the energy field from the shattering and fragmentation of separation, we piece ourselves back together, like pieces to a puzzle, to become whole and complete again.

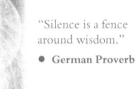

"Silence is a fence around wisdom."

- German Proverb

Repairing Our Auric Shields

The human aura has been damaged, invaded and violated during many lives of separation and disconnection. The aura appears to have fractures, cracks and leaks in the outer "eggshell" shield. As long as we are fragmented, we are vulnerable to outside astral violation and parasitic energy drains. This is actually very common, especially if there has been any abuse during early childhood.

And so we must liberate ourselves from the past history of violation and piece ourselves back together into whole human beings. To do so, we need to repair our auric shields, clean out the energetic invasion, and repair and mend all four levels of our being—the physical, the mental, the emotional and the spiritual bodies. This requires a concerted effort of dedication, discipline and loving self-care.

Step-by-step, we build a strong, impenetrable container of Light to house and protect Soul Presence within. I call this our Sacred Temple, and it is housed within the Chakra Pillar running through the center of our energy bodies. If you could picture in your mind—standing on a grounding platform anchored to the crystalline global grid under your feet, and Chakra Pillar of Light running up the center of the body all the way to your Higher Self and the Creator Source. This is the 12th Dimensional Pillar and Platform, the central infrastructure of our Light Body connected to all 12 dimensions of the Universe. Around the body, surrounding the human energy field is the Auric Shield, an energetic boundary surrounding the aura, like a crystal ball/orb of Light.

> "If you want children to keep their feet on the ground, put some responsibility on their shoulders."
>
> • Abigail Van Buren

Balancing Yin/Yang Energy

The human energy field is supported by the masculine energy on the right side of the body and the feminine energy on the left side, merging together in Sacred Union at the Heart Chakra.

The harmonious balance and integration of yin/yang energy is vital to maintaining a calm Core Center for the Soul to live in. The stillness at the connector point of yin and yang energy, is also called the Still-Point of balance. This is jeopardized by undue stress, fear and anxiety, abuse and violation—subsequently eliminating the vacuum effect of Core Energy and repelling the Soul Presence out of the body and into the Auric Field.

Not only do we need to pay attention to maintaining a balanced internal flow of yin/yang energy, but we also need to stay grounded in our bodies, in order to sustain the Still-Point field of Sacred Union. Well, I don't know about you, but achieving this constant state of still-point balance and union was very challenging for me.

For centuries past, humanity has been living in a dominant Patriarchal system, a world more disposed to brute force, male aggression and violence, linear mentality, and repressed emotions. The feminine principles of compassion, intuition, gratitude and artistic creativity have been diminished, demeaned or rejected. So it is no wonder that most human energy fields are overwhelmingly masculine, with a weak feminine. An integral part of the healing process is to run equally balanced yin/yang energy through our body/heart/mind, no matter what our birth gender. Obviously we need to surrender some of the harsher, controlling shadow masculine energy and embrace increasingly gentle, fluid intuitive feminine energy to blossom within. As we gradually restore the balanced flow of yin/yang energy, we begin to establish mutual receptivity between our inner masculine and feminine energies, thus establishing a balanced Still-Point Field for Soul Presence within. No longer do we need to seek outside ourselves for the opposite gender to "complete us." By maintaining whole, balanced yin/yang energy, we are evolving out of the co-dependent model of relationships.

Living in a Unified Field

Much will change in the coming years as we move away from Duality and the electromagnetic push/pull of opposing forces, and start living in unity consciousness. No more will we experience the opposite force pushing back at us as we try to manifest. In a Dualistic world of separation, all energy magnetizes the polar opposite to balance and complete itself. Positive needs negative, masculine needs feminine, Light needs Dark. Our mind is trained to expect one cannot exist without the polar opposite, as a complete set. In the world of Duality, "opposites attract" from the external world what is missing within due to polarity.

In a world of Unity Consciousness, all energy co-mingles in a harmonious field of existence—a Unified Field of Energy. Imagine positive particles and negative particles floating and bouncing around each other in a neutralized sea of interconnection. The Quantum Field blends the many particles of energy into a sea of unity consciousness, affecting the whole and interacting with each other. This field of wholeness has a unified resonance with all of nature, where "like magnetizes like" in co-existent harmony. When we connect to the Quantum Field, we enter a resonant particle field with our inner mind and feelings, magnetizing *matching* energy to materialize in form—"like attracts like." Within the Field of Oneness, we experience the full power and potential of the Law of Attraction!

> "To stay present in everyday life, it helps to be deeply rooted within yourself; otherwise, the mind, which has incredible momentum, will drag you along like a wild river."
>
> • Eckhart Tolle

It took some getting used to – this 5th dimensional field of wholeness! I found I was constantly bracing in anticipation of opposition whenever I initiated new manifestations. Duality had become so engrained in my being! But I eventually recognized through experimentation how the Law of Attraction can work outside of a polarized reality. My Soul inspired visions and new intuitive ideas, my heart swelled with magnetically charged Spiritual energy, and my chakras engaged with the quantum field of One-ness around me. I began to sense the matching energy to my visions in the Quantum Field, and so by utilizing the Quantum Vortex vacuum effect, I began to pull the matching energy within my Core. No longer plagued by counter-force, I was able to draw in my Soul's resources with the Law of Attraction from the quantum field of Unity Consciousness, now manifesting in form. As we shift into the 5D Field of Unity Consciousness, we start to dissolve the polarized magnetism from the body/heart/mind. We gradually materialize as floating particles of energy re-forming into a human body, flowing in the Cosmic Union of masculine/feminine, positive/negative, Light/Dark. We erase all memory of polarized separation and replace it with Unity Consciousness in every particle of our being.

Ending Co-Dependency

As we dissolve polarity from our cells and chakras, one of the areas to clear in our human lives will be co-dependency. Passed down at birth within the Family of Origin, the co-dependency patterning creates an external neediness for energy outside from others.. This creates interdependency on external sources and keeps us perpetually seeking external gratification.

"Thoughts crystallize into habit and habit solidifies into circumstances."

● Brian Adams

Oftentimes we have mistaken the magnetism of polarity, karmic contracts and co-dependency to be romantic Love. This is the farthest from the truth! We have become polarized beings in a planetary holographic reality of Duality and we cannot seem to understand that "opposites attract." This is actually the root of unsuccessful marriages and the destruction of romantic Love.

More often than not, we are charging our human electro-magnetic field with opposing forces. It stimulates an electrical charge in our Bio-Energetics and we feel "attracted" to the source of the charge ... convincing ourselves that it is Love. As long as we exist in the hologram of polarity, we cannot experience unconditional Love, for it only exists in a Field of Oneness. We need to become aware as human beings that electro-magnetic charge is not the energy of Love, but rather an electrical response in the codependent program of separation and karmic retribution.

The Need to Shield Our Energy

Sustaining and sourcing ourselves requires taking full responsibility, knowing that what we need resides within, and that we are designed to be nourished and fed by an abundant Universe. The programs of separation, disconnection and addiction have cross-wired our systems so we feel lacking and delinquent as co-dependent beings. When we split out of our Inner Core and reach outside ourselves to feed on other's energy, we are fragmenting ourselves, and attracting parasites to host on our energy. It cannot be avoided!

This operates similarly to moving into a new house. The outer boundaries of the home contain our personal belongings, just as our Auric Field contains our life force. In the case of the home, we lock the doors and windows at night to protect our belongings. Well, we should similarly be shielding our Human Energy Field to protect from parasitic invasion. When we leave our bodies, we have basically left our energy fields open and vulnerable to feeder lines or energy vampires. When we are under the controlling influence of victim-consciousness, we are constantly splitting outside ourselves to feed on external sources of energy, and leaving the doors wide open!

We need to create a strong, impenetrable auric Container—setting up energetic boundaries that protect, shield and contain our Divine life force within. When we leave our bodies and cannot maintain healthy boundaries, we suffer from energetic leaks (including guilt, shame, needy relationships or money drains), and we become vulnerable to outside attack or violation. It goes both ways—if we continue to consume external energy, then we are at risk of others consuming ours. It's a hard habit to break, but we must break free to evolve into Divine Humans.

I have to share something with you—this is what finally scared me to clean up my act. I took a long look at my own Auric Field and it appeared like Swiss cheese. When I realized that my needy, pulling behavior was weakening my energy field and leaving it vulnerable to invasion, I was motivated to stop my co-dependency. I started to become more discerning and selective in everything I participated in.

The key to success was determining whether other people, places and projects supported my personal boundaries or not.

Once I made the commitment to remain in my energetic container and source myself with the life force I needed, I also had to learn new behavior in setting personal boundaries. For many of us, we never were allowed to set personal boundaries as children. We were never allowed to say "NO" to prevent abusive violation to our personal space. I was raised in a family dynamic of co-dependent parents who were plugged right into my power center and living off my life force. I wasn't allowed to block their violation or energetic draining ... in fact, I was programmed to accept the invasion in order to earn their attention and approval.

Over time, we have developed distorted energy dynamics between family members, romantic couples, parents and children. It is pervasive and destructive to the very nature of our existence. We cannot maintain inner connection with Spirit when our energy fields are under constant attack. We must begin to clear out whatever invasion currently exists, denying access and cutting attachment chords to others. Next, we need to seal up our auric shields wherever there are holes, leaks and drains.

At that point, we have taken positive practical steps to create a secured energetic container, set strong personal boundaries and impenetrable auric shields, eliminate all energetic drains and invasion, and have committed to living as a self-sourcing Sovereign Being.

In summary, we must repair and rebuild our energetic container, not only to provide a "safety zone" for our human self to live in, but also to delineate and define personal boundaries and self-sovereignty.

Healing Exercise

As you move through the healing exercises to clear and heal all victim consciousness, you are gradually altering your life force upward into higher and purer frequencies. You begin to pulse in the expansive energy of crystalline light, sacred geometry and Soul Presence. While embodied in a human energy field you need to erect a strong, impenetrable container that provides a safe, inner sanctuary and shields you from external negativity. When living in an orb of crystal light you learn how to maintain personal space with integrity and self-care. This eliminates all behavior of pushing your energy on others or allowing violation to occur.

Sacred Geometry is the basic universal patterns of space, time and form that exist as the foundational design of everything in your reality. These symbols of geometry and mathematical ratios, harmonics and proportion are considered 'sacred' and found in nature, art, music, light, cosmology—the study of sacred geometry provides access and insights into the mysteries and laws of the Universe.

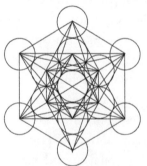

Sacred Geometry appears in the strands of DNA, in snow flakes, pine cones, flower petals, diamond crystals, the branching of trees, a nautilus shell, the galaxy you spiral within, the air you breathe—all life forms emerge from these sacred patterns.

The sacred geometry of the circle with "12 around 1" was said to emerge from the soul of the highest archangel of the Kabbalah, Lord Metatron. The cube represents the aesthetic properties and symmetry of the Platonic solids. As seen in alchemy, **Metatron's Cube** depicts the template of creational geometry and activates the phi spiral mathematics of the Quantum Vortex.

My Soul originates from the Metatron lineage, and activated Metatron's Cube in my energy field in 1997. We all seem to have an innate need to evolve and expand into ever greater fields of consciousness. Awakened conscious beings are like fractals evolving to ever greater scales of magnitude. Whenever you open the portal at your crown chakra to your higher self, you need to set up protection around your private space. I use this sacred invocation when activating the Quantum Vortex template:

INVOCATION FOR SACRED SPACE AND PROTECTION:

Place the chakra magnets on the bottom of the feet onto Gaia and your grounding platform at the base of your aura. Visualize stepping onto the Quantum Vortex template containing Metatron's sacred geometry, then secure your grounding platform onto the crystalline global grid. Visualize 12 pillars of light rising up from the 12 circles in Metatron's Cube sacred geometry, surrounding the body forming a sacred temple. Breathe deeply into the core of the body and proclaim the invocation:

"With the power of God/dess that I AM, I now speak the word to call forth my Divine Father and Divine Mother for their loving support. I call forth my own Divinity, my I Am Presence and breath my Soul Presence into my heart. I call forth Lord Metatron, Archangel Michael and all the Archangels and angelic realms, and to the of the High Priest, Melchizedek.

As I ground onto Gaia, I connect with Mother Nature, and call forth the Nature Kingdom, the Elementals and the Devic Realm and all the nature sprits of Gaia, to be present in this sacred space, to connect as one, to speak as one, to act as one. And I call forth the universal shields of crystalline light to wrap around me forming an Orb of Light for my protection and safety. And so it is."

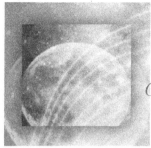

Chapter Ten

SOUL RETRIEVAL

As we reclaim our body/heart/mind from destructive external forces and build an inner connection with Spirit, we are intentionally moving into a more holistic union and higher energetic vibration. At this stage, we are actively clearing all mind-control programming and stored emotional pain from our being. This will activate a continual release of lower, denser energies from the mental, emotional and physical bodies. The denser energy will rise to the surface like oil on water—now incompatible with the higher vibration in the cells.

As the shadow disturbance works its way up to the surface for release, we become alert to a sense of discomfort and dis-ease. It may show up as physical symptoms, or emotional upset, or disturbing dreams, or addictive cravings ... the manifestation really depends on what the root of the disturbance is. However it appears, we will notice the disturbance and a feeling of imbalance. This signifies that an energetic healing crisis is occurring and that we need to get involved to accelerate the clearing. By tuning in, and paying attention to the constant condition within, we can transition through the purging process and regain balance as soon as possible.

It will require the power of our conscious mind to recognize the energetic disturbance as it comes to the surface, so we can guide and assist it out of our human energy field quickly. This involves the "Mind Over Matter" Principle, as we use the focused intention of the timeless mind to direct the movement of energy within our energetic field.

An Intention to Heal & Transform

As we become more familiar with navigating the flow of energy through our body, we can also focus our mind's intent on healing and transforming areas of imbalance. This is a gradual upgrade into mastering the way our body manifests life force or "chi," just like Chi Gong Masters . I have found that during this stage of Ascension, I was able to alter the actual form of energy with the images in my holographic mind/right brain. By focusing my attention on an image of total health and optimum functionality, I could initiate command code impulses from my mind to the receptor sites in my physical and emotional body.

> "If you want the whole thing, the gods will give it to you. But you must be ready for it."
> • Joseph Campbell

This activates the holistic approach to maintain a more comprehensive balance of health by recognizing all aspects of our being are becoming interrelated and connected. We can no longer separate our feelings or thoughts from the way our body is functioning, for they are now operating as one holistic being. We have evolved beyond the mechanical system of modern medicine that treats the body as a machine, and have entered the holistic world of interconnectivity where our body, mind and emotions flow together in constant communication and receptivity.

We begin to recognize that a symptom is a message that something is out of balance and needs corrective healing. The onslaught of a headache could be related to anxiety or undue emotional stress, the congestion in the lungs could be tied to grief or heartbreak. Degrading stomach disease is often caused by lack of inner nourishment ... and so on. By tuning into the physical symptom as a messenger for corrective action, we develop an internal knowing of our natural rhythms and requirements to maintain daily balance in our lives.

The Holographic Insert

Imagine the world stage as a holographic insert that camouflages the abundant Universe.

Not only does it block our ability to see and connect to our benevolent world, but it skews and distorts our perspective with fear and despair.

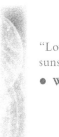

"Love comforteth like sunshine after rain."

● William Shakespeare

The holographic insert operates like stage scenery in a movie. It looks real, it feels real, and our mind is convinced it is the real world we live in. But it is an illusion of time and space, projected onto a blank movie screen, designed and manipulated to engage and evoke a response from the viewer. The scenery instills a certain timeline, a particlular century of human history. There are cultural and moral principles and belief systems embedded into the holographic projection. And all these images of the holographic insert flash within the movie projector of our subconscious minds—displaying this holographic environment out into the material world around us.

I didn't realize how prevalent the holographic insert was until I began to time-travel during past-life regressions. Once I could skip tracks and jump into parallel timelines, I was able to see the mechanism of holographic inserts so clearly. Each timeline had a specific "stage scenery" or hologram that was playing out a sample of the "victim-persecution" program. While I was remote-viewing the projected reality in that timeline, I empathically experienced the mental, emotional and physical responses to the staged holographic program. It sets up an entire blueprint of thoughts, feelings, and controlled behavior that successfully proliferates the debilitating karmic incarnational cycle.

The Soul Hologram

Once we realize that we are pulsing particles of energy forming into a particular blueprint·of visual imagery, we can begin to grasp the concept of projected holographic realities. I received instructions from my Higher Self on how to build a completely independent, sovereign Soul Hologram within my human energy field. In a series of steps, I was guided to create the energetic infrastructure, so I could exit the planetary simulation and live in my personal holographic reality. I began to "see" through the "eyes of the Soul."

The Quantum Vortex is a tool of alchemical transformation. By activating the crystallized sacred geometry, I was able to initiate the torque momentum around my being to spin in a Torus Vortex, creating the inner vacuum state stillness required for continual life force energy. In the same manner that ancient masters used the Arc of the Covenant (crystalline powered *phi* Spiral Vortex), I was able to recreate my own energy field into a newly formed Sovereign Soul Hologram, free of the Time Matrix simulation.

As we re-connect to our Soul essence and ancestral lineage, we activate the Soul Retrieval process. By adopting the Soul Hologram as our true authentic world reality, we establish an environment for Soul/body union to occur. We can imprint the nucleus of the cells with our Soul symbol or energetic signature like a fingerprint, the dynastic emblem of our Soul lineage. Rippling through the RNA, every cell in the body is marked with the Soul's family crest ... claiming the physical manifestation of our human biology as ours! It becomes an act of territorial ownership!

Addressing Past-Life Wounds

Now is a time of great celebration, as the inter-dimensional stagates open, unveiling the route to freedom and Soul Sovereignty. The collapsing veils remove the barrier of time and memory so that we can see, feel and integrate with the fragmented parts of our Souls that are still trapped in other timelines. This is often called the Soul Retrieval process, and may require active interception, karmic resolution and deep healing. Not only are we clearing shadow from this lifetime, but we also need to resolve and heal traumatized, soul fragments trapped frozen in time. As we piece ourselves back together into a whole being, we may find that we need to address wounded Soul aspects of past-life timelines.

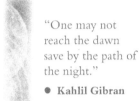

"One may not reach the dawn save by the path of the night."

• Kahlil Gibran

In *Mending the Past and Healing the Future with Soul Retrieval*, author, psychologist and medical anthropologist, Alberto Villoldo, shares an approach for entering timelessness to heal past events and correct your course toward your destiny. Villoldo discusses ways to heal yourself and your loved ones "by employing intention through practices used by shamans of the Americas—which, until now, have been inaccessible to most of the world. The shamans of old called this journeying."

It is through the Soul Retrieval process that we are able to journey into the Soul's timeless Unified Field, and according to Villoldo, "whatever we perceive is a projection of our inner world ... what we think of as the world of our imagination, the seers of old consider as real and tangible as our very physical world. To access the imaginal world, we need to enter into special states of consciousness that are very different from our ordinary daily consciousness. These are the states that have been cultivated by mystics, monks, saints, and yogis: it's the 'quiet mind' of the Laika and the Buddhas. This heightened awareness gives us access to our god-brain."

An example of this would be an irrational fear of drowning, loss of a loved-one, or childbirth. Many times, there exists past-life trauma involving physical harm or death that is still very charged and unresolved in the human consciousness. This requires rescuing the trapped Soul fragment to bridge across time and space, to return in union and merge with the Soul. I found that I had overwhelming fears of being a public figure, causing my body to shake and hyperventilate. My lungs would lock, throat close and my heart would surge with panic. I could barely breathe! Upon investigation, I uncovered past-life trauma stored in my psyche and cellular memory from false accusations and persecution, ending in violent deaths of burning at the stake or being beheaded. It was so powerful that I was gripped and frozen in fear, deeply affected by another timeline.

> "You become mature when you become the authority in your own life."
>
> • Joseph Campbell

The Soul Retrieval process allows people to resolve and release the stuck trauma, heal the original root cause, and integrate the lost Soul fragment. It is this final step that enables reclamation of all lost power that was stolen or destroyed during the parallel timeline. This is the final integration of our lost power!

Living Differently

By taking steps to move into the Soul Hologram and create the Sacred Temple or Soul Container, we proactively accelerate our capacity to ascend into becoming a Divine Human. As we feed our body crystallized Light and activate the Soul codes and templates, we are preparing our human biology to function as an enlightened being. Our days of feeling isolated and abandoned in the VOID are over! We become aware of the Quantum Field of all existence pulsing around us, supporting and sustaining our every need.

By erasing all barriers and veils to the Universal Field of Abundance, we begin to live very differently. At the onset, we must learn how to maneuver and function in a non-polarized environment ... letting go of old 3D habits such as using effort, Ego will, and hard work to manifest. These don't work in the Quantum Field, for we now must apply the principles of the true Law of One – "like attracts like." The more whole we become inside ... the more abundance is available to us in the Quantum Field. This applies to every area of our lives!

I have found that the more present I am in my body, in my heart and in my mind in the NOW, the more opportunities in life show up! I have become the Great Attractor! As I embody the Divine Energy of the Universe, the more I become a living, breathing magnet for Universal support. As I feed myself Divine Energy, I am in-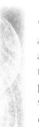

"Go placidly amid the noise and the haste, and remember what peace there is in silence."

● Max Ehrmann

haling particles of crystalline Light into the nucleus of my cells ... now vibrating with the pulse and rhythm of Universal creation. I have become ONE with All of Existence! This is not an esoteric proclamation ... but a real integration with the Quantum Field of All That Is. I now feel it pulse and flow inside and around my body! It's as if I'm moving in a fluid sea of energy that loves me and supports my needs. In another way, it's like living in the warm, caring, nourishing womb space of Creator God/Goddess.

As we become accustomed to living in this fluid field of pulsing Life, we begin to sense how our Soul needs to be expressed. This grows and forms within our heart and mind as ideas, desires, inspiration and motivation. The power of Divine Energy is birthing in our very Core and vibrating into the Quantum Field. It is at this point that we begin to create our lives as an artist engrossed in his masterpiece. Everything tingles and comes to life in the Quantum Field.

Our heart begins to swell with the fullness of Cosmic Unconditional Love ... we embody the sacred Love of God/Goddess. As our heart fills with the totality of yin/yang union, we begin to interact within the Quantum Field and live as a Divine Human.

The sacred geometry within the Cosmic Heart template (Vesica Pisces) resembles two inter-locking gold rings of Light. Once activated within the heart, it will energize the Field of Oneness with the Soul frequency in sacred union. The sacred geometry of the Cosmic Heart template invigorates the Quantum Field with our own heart magnetics. As we step into the Unified Field of Oneness, we become a human energy force field of creation.

---

*I*n summary, as we disentangle from the holographic reality of Duality, we must embrace and integrate all lost Soul fragments and piece ourselves back together to live as a Divine Human. The Soul Retrieval process of reintegration requires journeying into parallel timelines to heal the deeply seeded wounds of separation and absence of unconditional Love.

Healing Exercise

The Soul Retrieval process involves opening to all Soul timelines, incarnations, soul aspects and fragments – in order to integrate, blend and unify into Oneness. As you pull out of the dark web of the Time Matrix simulation, you are actively removing all presence of separation and disconnection to spirit. By consciously acknowledging and connecting to lost parts of your Soul, you can heal and release stuck trauma, resolve past karmic debt, fulfill and complete toxic soul contracts, and break free of the enslavement of Duality. In a very real way, you are piecing yourself back together from being shattered living in the Victim-Persecutor reality.

1. Using the 'Incarnational Wheel' analogy, the center Hub of the wheel represents the eternal Soul, also called the Over-Soul. All the spokes of the wheel represent every timeline your Soul has incarnated as an individualized Soul Aspect and the outer wheel symbolizes the container of your timeless Unified Field.
2. Initiate **Quantum Access™** and move into the upward *phi* spiral in the Quantum Vortex. By utilizing the counterclockwise spin of the Torus Vortex, you can swirl together all soul timelines and soul aspects/fragments into the heart center to merge with the OverSoul.
3. Within Zero Point energy of the vacuum state you can access the portal between the microcosm and the macrocosm, into the virtual particles of the Quantum Field – to all your past, present and un-manifested future potential!
4. Imagine all the spokes of the wheel (timelines) to dissolve into Divine Light, and merge every soul aspect into the central Hub of the Wheel – blending into the glorious sun of Soul Light!
5. During altered states of meditation your brain relaxes and expands to larger numbers of wave-lengths in the Zero Point Field, opening your right brain to awaken and receive new thought, visions and perceptions outside of the constraints of time.

In this expanded state your mind can wander the hallways of time in the Quantum Field and influence the possible outcome. With focused intention as the observer/influencer, your mind can pierce into the unformed anti-matter of space-time and set into motion a re-designed past or a newly formed future.

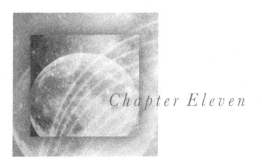

Chapter Eleven

A BRIDGE TO A NEW EARTH

TO RECAP, WE have been working step-by-step to build and activate the Soul's Light Container, and to also initiate the alchemical transformation of our cellular structure with crystalline photon light (silica)—from dense, carbon-based matter into becoming crystallized subatomic particles. We are training our mind and body to be fed and nourished on Love as our life force.

As we live in "observer consciousness," we become aware and focused on the thoughts, feelings and behaviors streaming through us, in order to clear, release and heal all programs of Ego-separation. This is an ongoing process as we discover layers and layers of deeply engrained patterning that were blocking or limiting our life potential. As we actively clear shadow energy and replace it with Divine Energy, we are gradually able to heal wounded Soul fragments, restore Soul Presence, and reclaim lost power.

The healing process also includes the resolution and regeneration of the wounded heart. The deep-seeded trauma of the "Fall of Man" and past history of "victim-persecution" has left a beaten and battered human heart. We are barely functioning, doing our best to engage with the world through a guarded, broken or frightened heart. We carry deep within our Core the Original Wound of Separation, which has left its mark—the debilitating grief and trauma of being severed from our connection to Divinity, our Soul Family, and the abundant Universe.

> "I don't know what your destiny will be, but one thing I do know: the only ones among you who will be really happy are those who have sought and found how to serve."
>
> • Albert Schweitzer

We can accelerate this healing process by spinning in the Quantum Vortex, taking detoxifying salt baths, receiving healing touch, nurturing massage and bodywork, reconnecting to Nature, and raising our energy frequency with meditative music and brainwave tones. All are benevolent acts of loving kindness and care for our human Spirit to recover, renew and rebirth inside.

At this stage of the Ascension Process, we begin to harmonize the human body, heart and mind with the unique vibration and rhythm of the Soul. By actively spinning in the Quantum Vortex, we are blending and integrating all levels of our being into holistic cohesion and coherence. This allows the mind to direct the flow of energy throughout all channels of the body, and proactively monitor and manage the balance of yin/yang energy in a stabilized order template.

All of these components are necessary in activating the Soul Hologram and intiating the Soul Retrieval process. A daily practice of meditation, yoga, breath-work, and walks in Nature will maintain an inner Still Point balance and peaceful calm. We are now living as a grounded, deeply present, conscious Divine Human!

Living Our Soul's Wisdom

Not only are we building the Soul-body-mind connection, but we are also learning how to protect our personal boundaries, preserve our Life Force energy and uphold the purity of our Soul Essence. We are finding our lost voice ... being able to communicate clearly what is acceptable behavior. As we discover where our energetic boundaries exist, we learn how to contain ourselves, to hold ourselves in check, not push our energy onto others.

"Hope is a waking dream."

● Aristotle

It may sound easy, but for most of us this requires an intuitive sense of where our energy ends and others begin. We are learning how to live in our Sacred Temple, merging in union with our Soul essence and speaking our authentic truth. The key to our success lies within the heart-brain, listening to inner guidance, following vibrational discernment, and building strong trust and faith with our higher wisdom.

I have witnessed many Spiritual seekers giving their power away to healers, gurus, channelers, False Ascension Masters, corrupted healing techniques, and so on. We must always remember that as long as anything exists in Duality, it contains shadow consciousness. By invoking other people or outside programs into our human energy field, we are jeopardizing our ascension process.

Since my Awakening 20 years ago, I was strictly guided by the High Council to avoid all Spiritual leaders, New Age channelings, and healing modalities that existed in Duality. I kept getting directed inward into the quiet stillness, to learn how to focus and listen to my superconscious mind. I would feel the touch of Spirit keep me in check, so I would resist reaching outside myself and give my personal power over to someone or something else. Well, it worked!

As I learned how to live in the present moment of Now, I was able to gradually train my mind to listen to the subtle messages—the higher frequencies of my Soul consciousness, wisdom and guidance. As I began to adapt to this new way of "listening" in the stillness, I also started to hear communication from my Higher Self about more planetary issues and the human Ascension Plan. All the while, I stayed contained in my Auric Field, strong protective shields up, and gradually merged my human self with Soul Presence into Oneness.

Raising Our Vibration

As we break free from the Time Matrix and reclaim our human energy field as our own, we can code the subatomic particles in our cells to pulse at the Soul's Divine frequency. We are increasing the physical body's frequency to come 'in phase' with the energy body's frequency. This is truly transformative! Our whole being takes on an entirely new and different energy. Not only do we feel a higher vibration inside, but our body and mind has access to a new frequency of consciousness. How we hold our body, our stance, and our presence is felt by all around us. We now emanate a powerful force field and radiate Soul consciousness around us.

It is the beginning of a new alignment not only with the Soul's natural vibration, but also with Universal rhythms. As we open our cells to hum and pulse in alignment with the rhythm of Nature, we begin to move in harmony within the Universal Field. We are in sync with the fluid motion of Creation. Our very being become a pulsing, thriving energy field of manifestation. Once the death code has been destabilized and removed, we can achieve molecular transformation by inserting into the nucleus of the cells an endless stream of photon wave particles. While spinning in the Quantum Vortex during deep meditation, we are able to breathe photon Light into the molecular level.

What is remarkable about utilizing photon wave/particles is that photons travel as bundles of Energy at the speed of Light. Despite the fact that a photon has no mass, it has velocity like a wave, and transfers consciousness to other particles. It is electrically neutral, at rest point, and perfectly identical to its anti-particle. And so, the amazing thing about photons is that they can travel into our polarized nuclear particles, stream balanced Energy into the molecular structure, and transfer Divine Intelligence into the cells.

An Incredible Opportunity

Due to the solar system's alignment with the Galactic Center, all life on Planet Earth is receiving an onslaught of photon wave particles from the gamma ray bursts in the black hole. In Gregg Braden's books, *Deep Truth* and *Fractal Time*, he explores the repetitive patterns or fractals in Nature as a model of repetitive cycles in human history. He offers insights about what we can expect beyond 2012, the completion of the Great World Age documented in the Mayan Calendar. Braden claims that "the conditions for 2012 have occurred in the past, that Earth's location in space triggers cycles of spiritual growth for humans, and that each cycle carries a window of opportunity—a choice point—that allows us to select a new outcome for the returning pattern!"

"The heart is like a garden. It can grow compassion or fear, resentment or love. What seeds will you plant there?"

● Jack Kornfield

We have within our grasp an astonishing abundance of Universal infusion of photon Light that our human biology can now metabolize. You may have noticed how everything is accelerating, time is speeding up and warping due to increasing Ascension waves. Scientists can measure the increase in Earth's frequency field, called the Shuman's Resonance, and tracking increasing solar flares contributing to climate change. According to *Science Daily* (March 20, 2009), scientists at Queen's University have made a discovery that could provide a deeper understanding about "the turbulent solar weather and its effect on our planet." Along with researchers at the University of Sheffield and California State University, they noticed "giant twisting waves in the lower atmosphere of the Sun. These huge twisting waves are evidence of a torsional structure in the plasma dynamics of the sun, a result of spacetime torque and Coriolis effects and the subsequent magnetic pole reversal."

"Let the beauty you love be what you do. There are thousands of ways we kneel and kiss the earth."

• Rumi

Due to the currently changing environment and quickening frequency, we have an incredible opportunity for a quantum leap in human consciousness. Not only can we transfer photon packets of Crystalline Light into the nucleus of our cells, but we can begin the process of transforming the very nature of how our cells manifest into form. This can be accomplished with Departicularization—a process of uniting a particle field of matter with an anti-particle field. In modern Particle Physics, when a sub-atomic particle and anti-particle collide, they annihilate each other in a burst of electromagnetic emissions. As we merge our particles with antiparticles within the vacuum state that exists at our Still Point in the Quantum Vortex, we can erase and release distortions. Electrons radiate or absorb energy in the form of photons when accelerated. During the Departicularization process, we can feed photon Light consciousness into the electrons that exist in the vacuum Zero Point Field. With the power of our holographic minds, we can recharge the atoms with newly coded electrons to chemically bond in newly forming physical matter. This allows our ability to reformulate our nuclear particle field into healthy, vibrant living human souls.

The Upward Spiral of Ascension

Our lower mind has been receiving incoming data streaming in from parallel timelines as we encounter the nuances of our Soul's essence and purpose. This information will continue to stream into conscious awareness so that we begin to actively alter the direction of our lives and meaningful pursuits. Look around you and witness how many people are shifting their career interests into service to healing and transformation.

The very essence of our DNA will continue to evolve into sub-atomic particles of quantifiable Light. Every packet of Light carries within it the history of our civilization, sparking alive the Original Human Blueprint. All we have to do is create the vacuum continuum that will propel our consciousness into the new reality. This bridge exists now, within our own DNA. By spinning in the torque momentum at Zero Point in the Quantum Vortex, the accelerated vibrational threshold or vacuum effect activates the codes held within the DNA to link up and create pathways of transference so that the body can become the living vessel of the Soul. It is the path of **Apotheosis**, or human ascension.

As our Energy reaches and touches the Quantum Field of all existence, we are able to peer into the parallel realities all around us. It begins to illuminate and shimmer in an alternate plane in our mind—across the thin membrane of time. The gateway to the 5th Dimensional Field has opened, allowing our consciousness to travel across the divide—out of Duality and into the Still-Point of present awareness. The '*New Earth*' author and teacher, Eckhart Tolle, claims "The foundation for a new earth is a new heaven – the awakened consciousness. The earth – external reality – is only its outer reflection."

As the mind enters the New 5D Earth hologram, we begin to access the purist Divine frequencies we've ever felt. They are free of polarized charge, purely neutralized energy waves that will feed us and restore healthy bodies. These 'New 5D Earth' energies are truly transformative in nature, catalyzing human genetics to upgrade and evolve into the full potential of Divine Humans.

Humanity is on accelerated trajectory into a new world of human evolutionary potential, unlike anything we've seen before!

Eventually, during our lifetime, our Human Energy Field will be pulsing with Love, the life force of the Universe. Our mind will become telepathic in nature, opening gateways of communication with other life forms. The illuminating Light will eliminate all hidden agendas, deceit and illusion from the earthly realm, for all shadow will be exposed in Pure Truth and witnessed. This will foster deeper authentic human connection and interaction, as we learn how to relate to each other in Truth and Love and form sustainable communities. The downward clockwise spiral of human decay and death will be eliminated, for we will have mastered the 3D emotions and dissolved time from our human biology. The 'New Earth' paradigm is riding in on the photon particle waves of universal intelligence from the Galactic Center. I invite you to join the upward spiral of Ascension into reclaiming your inherent lineage as a Divine Human.

In summary, we are living in extraordinary times, offering humanity an incredible opportunity to quantum leap into an ascending reality. As we transverse across the bridge of time, out of the Duality Matrix and into the Quantum Field of Unity Consciousness, we are being shown a New 5D Earth, a cooperative sustainable community of harmonious Love, living as Divine Humans!

Healing Exercise

As you move through the healing process and break free of Duality, you are liberating yourself to bridge across spacetime into the 5th Dimensional New Earth. Humanity has an extraordinary opportunity to quantum shift into a newly formed holographic reality of Unity Consciousness. Now at this momentous time you have at your disposal a quantum *"Life Tool"*, the Torus Quantum Vortex template...an ancient crystalline technology of transfiguration.

The hidden key to creation in our Universe occurs within the spiraling gravitational collapse inwards and electromagnetic expansion outwards in the standing wave pulse of **Singularity** in the Quantum Vortex phenomenon! There is growing astrophysical evidence that the vacuum structure found in galactic black holes also exists in the **Oscillating particles** at the *atomic scale level*.

The dynamic Universe emerges from **Singularity** in the constant motion of energetic collapse and expansion, continually recreating itself. Standing wave resonance is the natural pulse of life, like a cosmic heartbeat that fuels our Universe. The Pulse of Singularity in the Zero Point Field of the Quantum Vortex activates the DNA to awaken dormant codes of Unity Consciousness.

Quantum Access™ Healing Series

1. Unite all four levels into holistic health – mental, emotional, physical and spiritual.
2. Alter gravitational field to neutralize all polarity in the zero point vacuum state in Chakra Pillar. (heart and solar plexus).
3. Use the Quantum Vortex to spin and release all discordant patterns and programs of polarity from all four levels of the human energy field.

4. Enter the timeless vacuum state in the Quantum Vortex to repair, mend and resolve all past trauma, wounds, and karmic contracts.
5. Clear the emotional pain body of all truama.
6. Heal the Original Wound of Separation from early childhood mend, repair and rebirth inner child psyche.
7. Mend and integrate the fragmented self.
8. Stairstep the descending Soul into the human body/heart center to become Whole again.
9. Activate the Light Body – electrical current of Spirit (kundalini) in the bio-circuitry of the body.
10. Transform human DNA and convert from carbon-6 molecules to crystalized carbon-7 molecules.
11. Access All Time—open channel to all 12 dimensions of spacetime to access Total Recall—the Soul wisdom, knowledge, skills, and abilities from the ages.
12. Transition from Ego will and control to living Soul purpose according to Divine Will.

Quantum Access™ is your tool to fuel your energy field in the standing scalar wave pulse with continual Life Force! As you pull out of the dark Matirx of Duality, you step into the eternal, infinite source of cosmic life force emanating from the Quantum Field. The New Earth is waiting for you...

SACRED SYMBOLS

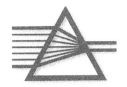

Light

Light is seen as the fundamental source of all matter, the spark of Creation, that transfers divine intelligence and the love and wisdom radiating from God.

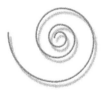

Spiral

The Spiral is the ancient symbol of the goddess, the womb, fertility, continual change, and the evolution of the universe. A logarithmic spiral or *Phi* spiral grows in a geometric expansion as self-similar fractals with increasing distance from the center. It often appears in nature (snail, shells, DNA, galaxy).

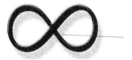

Infiinity

In ancient India and Tibet, the Infinity symbol represented perfection, dualism, and unity between male and female. It also represents equilibrium or the balance of various forces, and has become a secular mathematical symbol for infinity in numbers, time or space (eternity).

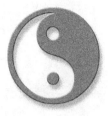

The Tao (Yin Yang)

An ancient Chinese symbol used originally to represent a widespread belief in unity, polarity, holism. Harmony is achieved when the two are perfectly united and balanced: positive/negative, light/ dark, male/female, etc. Yin is the dark, passive, negative female principle. Yang is the light, active, positive masculine principle. Since the balance between yin and yang is dynamic and constantly changing, the symbol represents the blending of opposing energies at the heart of Holistic Health.

All-Seeing Eye

A universal symbol representing multi-dimensional intuitive sight, inner vision, higher knowledge. In eastern traditions the Third Eye in the forehead symbolizes enhanced perception directed inwards in meditation. In Freemasonry the Eye in the capstone of the Pyramid is a mystical image demonstrating the omniscient (all-knowing) God and eternal justice. The opening of the eye, in metaphysical teachings, symbolizes a time of awakening, the evolution of consciousness, and the activation of the pineal gland to attain multi-dimensional sight.

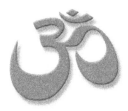

Om

Sanskrit letters or symbol for the "sacred" Hindu sound OM (Ohm or Aum) is found in Sikh theology as a symbol of God. The sacred tone represents the manifestation of the divine as the first original vibration of creation, without beginning or end, it embraces all of existence. In essence, *OM* or *Aum* is the united harmonic tones of all 12 sound waves from all 12 dimensions of spacetime.

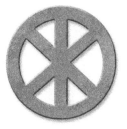

The Wheel

A universal symbol of cosmic unity, astrology, movement, the sun, the zodiac, karmic cycle of reincarnation, and earth's cycles of renewal and evolution. In Soul Retrieval, the sacred circle plus the radiating spokes form the wheel. The central hub of the wheel represents the OverSoul and the spokes signify the multiple timelines.

SACRED GEOMETRY

Sacred Geometry has evolved from the belief that basic universal patterns of space, time and form exist as the foundational design of everything in our reality. According to this viewpoint these symbols of geometry and mathematical ratios, harmonics and proportion are 'sacred'. Found in nature, art, music, light, cosmology – the study of sacred geometry provides access and insights into the mysteries, and laws of the Universe.

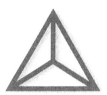

Tetrahedron: As the most stable regular solid figure, it is most easily recognized as a Pyramid with a triangular base. In western hermetic tradition, the square base represents earth, matter, form and manifestation: the upward movement to the point representing heaven and human enlightenment. Tetrahedrons are also the basic foundation for crystal silicate structures, and fundamental to the transformation of cellular composition from dense matter to crystal (silicon) light.

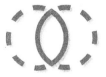

Vesica piscis: One of the simplest forms of sacred geometry, the shape is the intersection of two circles with the same radius. Often called the symbol of fusion or Sacred Union, it represents the interactions and interdependence of opposing forces uniting, as well as the sacred marriage of Twin Flame energy.

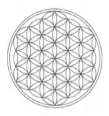

The Flower of Life: The geometrical figure composed of multiple evenly spaced, overlapping circles (including the Vesica Piscis), that are arranged so that they form a flower-like pattern with a sixfold symmetry like a hexagon. It is considered a sacred template of Creation, for which all life springs; believed to contain the Akashic Records of universal truth of all living things.

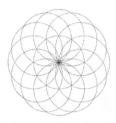

Tube Torus: The sacred geometry of the Tube Torus contains Vortex Mathematics that engages light and gravitational fields according to the universal Akashic Records. If two or more different types of energy cross or meet, and they are not compatible or sympathetic with each other, they will begin to turn upon each other in a rotating and spiral motion. This toroidal form will continue until one absorbs and cancels the other out, or they become so equally balanced the rotating can go on indefinitely.

Zero Point (Still Point): The spiraling symbol of Sacred Geometry depicting the creational force (DNA) found in a central vacuum dynamic within a Black Hole or Torus Vortex that produces a zero gravity field. Now considered a powerful potential of energy source, the Zero Point exists as the portal to the Quantum Field which souls enter to experience linear time. Activated within the source of creation, the human DNA genetic programming is coded to remember all at Zero Point (Enlightenment).

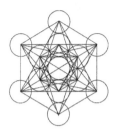

Metatron's Cube: In early Kabbalist scriptures the sacred geometry of this cube was said to emerge from the soul of the highest archangel of the Kabbalah, Metatron. The cube delineates the aesthetic properties and symmetry of the Platonic solids and the double star tetrahedron Merkaba. As seen in alchemy, Metatron's Cube depicts the crystalline template of 12 Dimensional creational geometry vortex mathematics..

Golden Ration of *Phi* (φ): Also known as the golden mean or divine proportion, *phi* depicts the natural aesthetic and balance between symmetry and asymmetry that expresses an underlying truth about existence. Scientists see the same geometric and mathematical patterns as the Golden Ratio arising directly from natural principles. The Golden Ratio is often denoted by the Greek letter phi, usually lower case (φ). The first known approximation of the golden ratio by a decimal fraction, stated as "about 0.6180340."

$$\varphi = \frac{1 + \sqrt{5}}{2} = 1.6180339887...$$

Leonardo da Vinci studied sacred geometry and its mathematical properties, and used the Golden Ratio of *phi* in his artwork...as seen in the cultural icon, the Vitruvian Man.

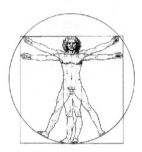

The study of geometric relationships to wave interaction (sound) can be traced back to the Greek philosopher and mathematician, Pythagoras. He discovered that musical notes could be translated into mathematical equations and believed this gave music powers of healing, as it could "harmonize" the out-of-balance body. In this manner, the sacred geometry of universal harmonic toning activates the alignment and manifestation of a Zero Point Field within the vacuum state of the Quantum Vortex.

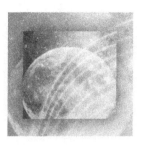

GLOSSARY

3rd Eye Chakra – Human Energy Center associated with the Pineal gland in the geometric center of the brain. When activated the 'intuitive eye' has increased psychic awareness, inner visions and connection to the holographic mind.

12 Pillars of Light – The 12 around 1 sacred pattern of a 12th Dimensional Universe can be found in our clocks, zodiac, alchemy wheel, mandalas and archetypes of sovereignty and divinity (Greco-Roman Temples). The Quantum Vortex Activations ignite the 12 Pillars of Light to rise, tone and spin upward from the sacred geometry of Metatron's Cube.

Anti-Particle Field – According to Quantum Field Theory, most kinds of particles have a corresponding anti-particle with the same mass and opposite electrical charge. The virtual-particle field is the non-physical, unmanifested potential of creation.

Auric Field – A field of subtle, luminous radiation emmanating from and surrounding a person or object, in multiple etheric layers of vibrational range attributed to the mental, emotional and spiritual bodies.

Auric Shield – The outermost layer surrounding the Auric Field, somewhat like an egg-shell shape, creating an energetic container around the human energy field.

Bio-Energetics – Universal energy principles of biological systems found in Biochemistry that studies the energy flow through living systems, including cellular processes and respiration, metabolic processes, and the production and utilization of intracellular energy transfer. The foundational principle based on the holistic model of living beings – the interconnectedness of an energetic body and a physical body.

Central Core – Internal space, gravitational center of human energy field– comprised of the heart and solar plexus as the Order Matrix.

Core Pillar – Main central Chakra column of the Energetic Body.

Corrupted Codes – Distorted reptilian hybrid genetic codes blocking or corrupting the Original Human Blueprint that were inserted during genetic re-engineering.

Crystalline Light – Photon light particles of silicate crystal compounds with tetrahedron formations – when metabolized will transform carbonized density into crystalline light within the cellular structure.

Death Code – Distorted consciousness code to devolve the human life source to decay, age and die in the repeated clockwise incarnational karmic cycle.

Divine Human – Fully evolved, ascended 12th Dimensional actualized human Soul.

Divine Light – Highest vibrational 12th Dimensional Light of pure truth in crystalline structure.

Divine Soul – Original God Spark of creation, the I AM Presence actualized with unique energetic signature.

Crystalline Global Grid – overlay network of crystal light pathways in the surface of the earth for human souls to connect and ground their human energy field onto.

Ego Identity – False human persona developed by the ego self.

Frequency of Phi – see index for Sacred Geometry.

God Light – The purist elemental source of Creator, encompasses the entire spectrum of light (Monad).

God Seed Code – The genetic code required for the human bioenergetic system to metabolize Divine Light at the cellular level.

Glossary

Golden Ratio – see index for Sacred Geometry.

Indigo Light – From the spectrum of Light the color/tone of Indigo, origin is Sirian Light, and utilized in healing and neutralizing polarized, magnetic charge.

Master Receptor Cell – Located in the pineal crystals, the MRC is the hologram of the entire biology, the main command-code designator for the entire Bio-Energetic genetic blueprint.

Mind Matrix – An embedded array or grid which streams repeated patterns of programmed beliefs, behaviors and subconscious thought forms that create a controlled, polarizing holographic reality. Originates from the planetary enslavement program and feeds into the primal reptilian brain stem.

New Earth Hologram – An alternate 5th Dimensional holographic reality constructed for the inner mind to access through unity consciousness.

Particle Field – According to Quantum Field Theory, the particle field is the time/space continuum of Creation manifested in the 3rd Dimensional material world, (sub-atomic particles) existing as matter.

Photon Light – In physics, a photon in an elementary particle, the force carrier of the electromagnetic field and the basic "unit" of light and all other forms of electromagnetic radiation (eg. Lasers). Universal intelligence travels in photon light.

Pineal Crystal Seed – Upon kundalini activation the dormant pineal 'antenna' residing in the energetic body opens multi-dimensional psychic awareness.

Separation – The divisive program to 'separate' and alienate the Soul from the human Bio-Energetic system, as well as the ego-mind from the collective field of consciousness.

Soul Dynastic Lineage – The timeless Soul's origin of creation, home star-system and family dynasty – some Souls originate with Earth, and others originate from a parallel universe or star system.

Soul Hologram – An independent, sovereign holographic reality (container) reflecting the authentic, original blueprint of Soul essence, purpose and energetic signature.

Soul Union – The term applied to the unification of the Soul and Human self in Oneness – one singular, united, holistic living being.

Super-Conscious Mind – The Higher Mind's quantum awareness outside of the limits of time/space that can access the timeless 12 Dimensions of Universal Intelligence.

Quantum Vortex template – Crystalline-based Vortex technology coded in a sacred geometry template for human activation.

Quantum Access™ – Developed by Meg Benedicte. Series of 12 Dimensional energetic activations in the Quantum Vortex to eradicate polarity, separation and enslavement Matrix, as well as ignite the Soul's Merkaba for human ascension. The Quantum Vortex Activations are the most effective, accelerated method to unlock trapped emotional/mental/chemical information from the cells by neutralizing the gravitational field of Duality.

Universal Harmonics (the Sacred Tones of Creation) – entire light/tone spectrum of 12 dimensions used to attune with universal order, balance and harmony within the Quantum Vortex – utilized to stabilize and establish a vacuum state of Still Point connection to the quantum field of all creation.

Vacuum effect – The vacuum continuum is defined as the state with no particle or antiparticle – zero gravitational state existing at the zero Point in Black Hole (Torus Vortex) dynamics.

Violet Ray of Sovereignty – The 7th dimensional Ray of the color light/tone spectrum – Violet light infuses mercy and forgivenss, and resonates with the energy of Freedom, liberty and sovereignty.

Yin/Yang Balance – see index for Sacred Geometry

Zero Point Field – see index for Sacred Geometry

Web of Duality – Interlocking matrix or web of shadow consciousness permeating the holographic realm of Duality.

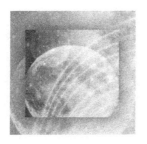

REFERENCES

Gregg Braden, *Fractal Time*, New York, New York, Hay House, Inc. 2010

Gregg Braden, *The Divine Matrix*, New York, New York, Hay House, Inc. 2008

Gregg Braden, *Deep Truth*, New York, New York, Hay House, Inc. 2012

Courtney Brown, Ph.D., *Cosmic Voyage*, New York, New York, The Penguin Group, 1996

Rhonda Byrne, *The Secret*, New York, New York, Three Rivers Press, 1998.

Deepak Chopra, *Ageless Body, Timeless Mind*, New York, New York, Three Rivers Press, 1998.

Barbara Hand Clow, *The Mayan Code: Time Acceleration and Awakening the World Mind*, Rochester, Vermont, Inner Traditions/Bear & Company, 2007

Dr. Masaru Emoto, *The Hidden Messages in Water*, Hillsboro Oregon, Beyond Words Publishing Inc. 2004.

Debbie Ford, *The Dark Side of the Light Chasers*, New York, New York, Riverhead Books, 1998.

Ken Keys, Jr., *The Hundredth Monkey*, Camarillo, CA Devorss & Co., 1984.

Lynne McTaggart, *The Field: The Quest for the Secret Force of the Universe*, New York, New York, HarperCollins Publisher, 2001.

Lynne McTaggart, *The Intention Experiment: Using Your Thoughts to Change Your Life and the World*, New York, New York, Free Press, Simon & Schuster Inc., 2008.

James Van Praagh, *Talking to Heaven*, New York, New York, Penguin Books, 1997.

Rowena & Rupert Shepherd, *1000 Symbols*, New York, New York, Thames & Hudson, Inc., 2002.

Eckhart Tolle, *The Power of Now*, Novato, California; New World Library, 1999.

Eckhart Tolle, *A New Earth*, New York, New York, Hay House, 2006.

Alberto Villoldo, Ph.D., *The Four Insights: Wisdom, Power and Grace of the Earthkeepers*, New York, New York, Hay House 2006.

Alberto Villoldo, Ph.D., *Mending the Past and Healing the Future with Soul Retrieval*, New York, New York, Hay House, 2005.

Brian L. Weiss, M.D., *Many Lives, Many Master*, New York, New York, A Fireside Book, 1988.

Fred Alan Wolf, Ph.D., *The Yoga of Time Travel: How the Mind Can Defeat Time*, Wheaton, IL, Quest Books, 2004.

Katherine Woodward Thomas, *Calling in the One*, New York, New York, Three Rivers Press, 2004.

Nassim Haramein, Director of Research, The Resonance Project, *Schwarzschild Proton paper, Crossing the Event Horizon* DVD, www.theresonanceproject.org, *The Science of Oneness*, www.consciousmedianetwork.com

The Bible, Book of Genesis, New Revised Standard Version Ellie Crystal, Sacred Geometry, www.crystalinks.com

Science Daily, Top Science News, www.sciencedaily.com (March 20, 2009). Wikipedia, www.wikipedia.com

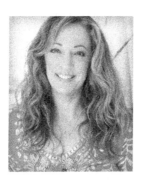

ABOUT THE AUTHOR

Meg Benedicte, author, teacher, Quantum Healer, and founder of Quantum Access™, is an expert in treating the root cause of human dysfunction, unrealized potential and spiritual disconnection.

In 1994, Meg experienced a profound awakening that activated her inherent template for utilizing the Quantum Vortex as a powerful tool for transformation. Through extensive research in Bio-Energetics and Quantum Healing, Meg discovered the magnitude of change possible when tapping into the Zero Point Field of vortex energy. According to research physicists, the spinning Torus Vortex provides access to a continuum of universal energy.

With this transformational quantum technique, Meg Benedicte can access crystallized Light to eradicate disease, polarity and the decomposition of time. She helps clients to quickly shift consciousness, unlock karma and remove energetic patterns so they can clear out-of-date 3D systems that limit their human experience. By utilizing sacred geometry and *Phi* Harmonics to enhance wave inter-action, she developed the powerful Quantum Access™ technique, that is coded to bend space, unlock gravity, access the 5th Dimension and activate Soul DNA / divine Light Body.

Meg Benedicte has been sharing these dramatic findings in her proprietary process Quantum Access™ private practice, in the Quantum Access™ Training Courses, with global audiences in telecasts/webinars, various speaking events, her online radio show podcasts at blogtalkradio.com/newearthcentrall, the Dr. Pat Show, World Puja Show, Transformation Talk Radio and Global Meditation Broadcasts.

You can visit Meg at:
www.newearthcentral.com
www.quantumaccess.org

CPSIA information can be obtained
at www.ICGtesting.com
Printed in the USA
LVHW110158080520
655210LV00005B/1460